Baillière's

CLINICAL
OBSTETRICS
AND
GYNAECOLOGY

INTERNATIONAL PRACTICE AND RESEARCH

Baillière's

CLINICAL
OBSTETRICS
AND
GYNAECOLOGY

INTERNATIONAL PRACTICE AND RESEARCH

Volume 2/Number 2
June 1988

Gynaecology in the Elderly

STUART L. STANTON FRCS, FRCOG
Guest Editor

Baillière Tindall
London Philadelphia Sydney Tokyo Toronto

Baillière Tindall 24–28 Oval Road
W.B. Saunders London NW1 7DX

The Curtis Center, Independence Square West
Philadelphia, PA 19106–3399, USA

1 Goldthorne Avenue
Toronto, Ontario M8Z 5T9, Canada

Harcourt Brace Jovanovich Group (Australia) Pty Ltd
32–52 Smidmore Street, Marrickville, NSW 2204, Australia

Exclusive Agent in Japan:
Maruzen Co. Ltd. (Journals Division)
3–10 Nihonbashi 2-chome, Chuo-ku, Tokyo 103, Japan

ISSN 0950–3552

ISBN 0–7020–1301–3 (single copy)

Baillière's Clinical Obstetrics and Gynaecology is published four times each year by Baillière Tindall. Annual subscription prices are:

TERRITORY	ANNUAL SUBSCRIPTION	SINGLE ISSUE
1. UK & Republic of Ireland	£35.00 post free	£15.00 post free
2. USA & Canada	US$68.00 post free	US$25.00 post free
3. All other countries	£45.00 post free	£18.50 post free

The editor of this publication is Seán Duggan, Baillière Tindall, 24–28 Oval Road, London NW1 7DX.

Baillière's Clinical Obstetrics and Gynaecology was published from 1983 to 1986 as *Clinics in Obstetrics and Gynaecology*.

Typeset by Phoenix Photosetting, Chatham.
Printed and bound in Great Britain by Mackays of Chatham PLC, Chatham, Kent.

Contributors to this issue

MARK BRINCAT PhD, MRCOG, Senior Registrar, St. George's Hospital, Blackshaw Road, London SW17 0QT, UK.

CHRISTOPHER HUDSON MChir, FRCS, FRCOG, FRACOG, Consultant Gynaecologist, St Bartholomew's Hospital, West Smithfield, London EC1A 7BE, UK.

JOHN KELLETT MB, FRCP, FRCPsych, St. George's Hospital Medical School, Department of Geriatric Medicine, Jenner Wing, Cranmer Terrace, London SW17 0RE, UK.

JAMES MALONE-LEE MBBS, MRCP, Senior Clinical Lecturer, Academic Department of Geriatric Medicine, University College and Middlesex School of Medicine, St. Pancras Hospital, St. Pancras Way, London NW1 0PE, UK.

PETER H. MILLARD MBBS, FRCP, Eleanor Peel Professor, Geriatric Teaching and Research Unit, St. George's Hospital Medical School, Cranmer Terrace, London SW17 0RE, UK.

C. MARJORIE RIDLEY MA, BM, BCh, FRCP, Consultant Dermatologist, Elizabeth Garrett Anderson Hospital, 144 Euston Road, London NW1; Royal Northern Hospital, Holloway Road, London N7; Whittington Hospital, St. Mary's Wing, Highgate Hill, London N19 5NS, UK.

ANTHONY G. RUDD MA, MB, BChir, MRCP, Lecturer, Department of Geriatric Medicine, St. George's Hospital, Cranmer Terrace, London SW17 0RE; Consultant Physician for the Elderly, St. Thomas Hospital, Lambeth Palace Road, London SE1, UK.

DAVID GWYN SEYMOUR BSc, MD, MRCP, Senior Lecturer in Geriatric Medicine, University of Wales College of Medicine, Cardiff Royal Infirmary (West Wing), Newport Road, Cardiff CF2 1SZ, UK.

STUART L. STANTON FRCS, FRCOG, Urodynamic Unit, Department of Obstetrics and Gynaecology, St. George's Hospital Medical School, Lanesborough Wing, Cranmer Terrace, London SW17 0RE, UK.

JOHN W. W. STUDD MD, FRCOG, Consultant Obstetrician and Gynaecologist, King's College Hospital, Denmark Hill, London SE5, UK.

HARVEY WAGMAN MBBS, FRCSEd, FRCOG, Consultant in Obstetrics and Gynaecology, Barnet General Hospital, Wellhouse Lane, Barnet, Herts EN4 3DJ, UK.

DAVID WARRELL MD, FRCOG, Consultant Gynaecologist, St Mary's Hospital, Whitworth Park, Manchester M13 0JH; Clinical Lecturer, University of Manchester, Medical School, Oxford Road, Manchester M13 9PT, UK.

Table of contents

FORTHCOMING ISSUES

Foreword

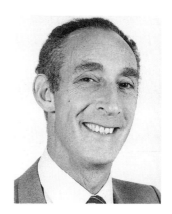

'Cease to fume at destiny' (Marcus Aurelius) is the anti-quote which sums up the purpose of this book—an attempt to recognize and treat disease in the elderly and not to accept them as a consequence of growing old and thereby summarily dismiss them.

The elderly are an important and neglected group of patients. They form 15% of the population, which will rise to 19% by the year 2025. Despite our growing awareness of their needs, they are still not expected by many to enjoy sexual fulfilment, urinary continence or qualify for elective surgery.

This volume attempts to show that, whilst they are entitled to this and more, there are ageing changes which may alter the presentation of disease and confer a higher risk for surgery. The choice of contributors emphasises the close links we need with colleagues in different specialities, to provide the best care for our elderly.

The first two chapters discuss the ageing process, its implications and pathophysiology. The preparation of the patient for surgery, her expectations, the operative and post operative morbidity and mortality, are dealt with in Chapter 3. The pathophysiology and symptoms of the menopause, the arguments for and against hormone replacement therapy and its routes of administration, are critically reviewed by Mark Brincat and John Studd, and illustrate that some important components of the ageing process can at least be delayed.

Vulval lesions, an important source of patient distress, are reviewed by Marjorie Ridley. Urinary incontinence, the fear of many younger women and the ignoble reason given by some institutions for refusing admission to the elderly, is discussed by James Malone-Lee. In the chapters on post menopausal bleeding and cancer, the strategies for management in the elderly are reviewed.

Sexuality in the elderly has always been a taboo subject, with many treating this with embarrassment or disbelief. John Kellett sensitively discusses the issues and how they should be managed.

Finally prolapse; and here only a plea, similar to that in other chapters, that ultimately age should not be a bar to surgery. Rather it is primarily the patient's fitness and the need to preserve her independence and dignity which are important.

I should like to thank Tricia Black, my research assistant, for her patience and skill in assisting in the editorship of this volume—an ageing process in itself—and acknowledge Seán Duggan and Margaret Macdonald, of Baillière Tindall, for their enthusiasm and support for this book.

S. L. STANTON

Dedication

To my mother, Sarah Stanton, whom I watched move courageously from middle to older years.

1

What is ageing?

ANTHONY G. RUDD
PETER H. MILLARD

INTRODUCTION

The only certainty in life is that within a finite space of time it will end. At the biological level this is important to permit evolutionary changes to occur within the species; in the shorter term it has perhaps greater implications for evolution of society. The knowledge of man's mortality must have been welcome many times throughout history, faced with tyrants or corrupt government. It is only since the beginning of this century that the life expectancy of man has exceeded 50 years in developed countries; the problems associated with an ageing society, particularly the provision of health care has been highlighted with recent debates about funding. An understanding of the mechanisms and consequences of normal ageing and of the differences in disease patterns in the elderly are essential to maintain fitness in this group of individuals and thereby reduce dependency.

DEFINITIONS

Ageing

We grow oldest fastest when youngest

The definitions of ageing can broadly be divided into two groups; those that view ageing as part of the continuum of development, biomorphis, occurring as an inevitable consequence of the processes of growth and maturation and therefore inseparable from them and those viewing ageing as a separate event occurring in the late stages of life concerning only degenerative processes and functional decline. The difficulty in defining ageing leads to problems in assessing the results of experimental work. An old mouse to one research scientist may not mean the same to another; different species age in different ways and there are often considerable interstrain variations. Time is not the only factor. We all know of individuals who look younger than their years and people who appear to age rapidly. We have no difficulty in recognizing an old house or piece of furniture. It may not be so obvious with complex multicellular organisms. As old furniture can be made to look young, so some people try to put off the signs of the passage of time by plastic surgery and expensive cosmetics.

Longevity

Longevity means literally a long duration of existence. It is used to define the maximum duration of life and is species-specific. Thus the Mayfly will not live longer than 24 hours, the fruit fly 75 days and man 120 years. Despite significant advances in medicine and improvements in living conditions the longevity of man has not changed. Greater proportions of the population, however, are living to ages approaching their biological maximum.

Lifespan

This is a statistically derived calculation of the future duration of life derived from actuarial data. Formulae have been devised, the best known of which is the Gompertz equation first published in 1825:

$$L_x = d\,(g)^{Qx}$$

where d, g and Q are constants characteristic of each population and L_x is the number of persons living to age x.

Senile

This means old. It is a term frequently misused to mean old and stupid. The best definition perhaps is that senility means older than the examining doctor!

DEMOGRAPHY

Not only are the absolute numbers of elderly people increasing in industrial countries but the proportion of old to young is also increasing. These changes have been described by Butler (1979) as 'the greying of nations'. In 1900 between 2.5 and 3.0% of the world's population was over 60 years of age. Now approximately 8.5% are over 60 years. In the United Kingdom in 1986, 15.3% of the population were over 65 years with 1.2% over 85 years. It is projected that by the year 2025, 18.8% will be over 65 and 2.3% over 85. The UK now has the largest proportion of the population aged 60 years or over in the European Community. Estimated population trends are summarized in Figure 1.

To understand the reasons for these changes one must look both at birth rates and childhood mortality as well as any changes that may have occurred in the old themselves: 'To live to be old one must not die young'.

Birthrates

To maintain a constant population in a developed society every woman

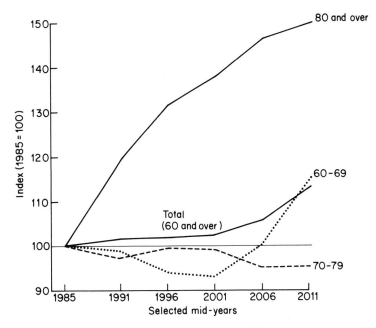

Figure 1. Projected changes in the population, 1985 to 2011. From Thompson (1987).

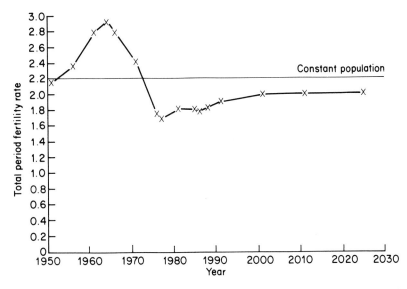

Figure 2. The actual and predicted average number of children born per woman throughout their child-bearing lifespan. From the Office of Population Censuses and Statistics.

should have 2.2 children during the course of her lifetime. A figure higher than this will lead to an expanding population and lower will result in a decline

Using data such as this (Figure 2) projections can be made of the age distribution of the population well into the next century. Thus the baby boom of the early 1960s will lead to a 'geriatric' boom in 2030.

Infant mortality

In the eighteenth century half of all live-born children died before their fourteenth birthday. In some parts of the world infant mortality remains at these appallingly high levels. By 1961 this had fallen in the UK to 23.4 per 1000 live births and has further declined to 10.1 per 1000 in 1986. The most dramatic fall has been in the death rates of children under one year, being 149 per 1000 in 1840, 22.05 per 1000 in 1961 and 9.5 per 1000 in 1986. The reasons for the decline include: better nutrition for both the pregnant mother and young child; better standards of obstetric care; control of the water and sewerage system leading to improved hygiene; and immunization and antibiotics, virtually eliminating lethal infections in childhood.

Death rates in the elderly

The expectation of life of an 80-year-old has risen little this century; in 1906 it was 5.4 years for a female; by 1961 this had risen to 6.3 years and by 1984, 7.6 years. The death rate of the 75–84 year age group fell between 1961 and 1986 from 89.1 per 1000 to 63.2 per 1000 for females. Again the reasons for the apparent improvement in health are multifactorial and it is probably the detection and treatment of diseases earlier in life rather than any direct impact on the health of the elderly that has influenced the figures.

Expectation of life

It can be seen from Figure 3 that it is only this century that the mean life expectancy at birth exceeded that of the mean age of the menopause. Many of the problems being discussed in this book have therefore only been common this century.

Male: female differences in lifespan

From the moment of conception males have a higher mortality than females, with differences in life expectancy of 5.9 years at birth and a ratio of females to males of 1.8:1 over the age of 75 years. The superiority of females over males is not confined to man; there is evidence that it is to be found in the majority of animal species including relatively simple life forms such as the housefly (Rockstein and Lieberman, 1958). A few species of birds and reptiles, however, have longer-living males than females. A frequent feature is that the shorter living sex is the one with the XY chromosome combination: perhaps recessive alleles on the X chromosome act to the

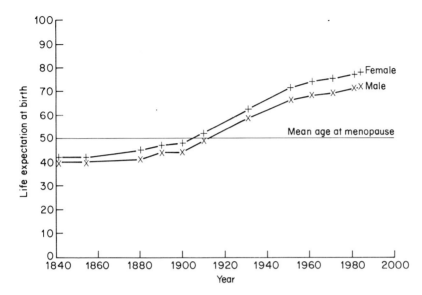

Figure 3. Life expectancy at birth, 1840–1986. Only since 1900 has the mean life expectancy exceeded the mean age of the menopause. From the Office of Population Censuses and Statistics.

detriment of the individual for which there are no counteracting alleles on the Y chromosone (Bellamy, 1985). Alternatively the differences in endocrine status may be important. Males castrated before puberty increase their life expectancy when compared to post-pubertal castration (Hamilton and Mestler, 1969). How much influence cigarette smoking, work patterns, alcohol and other social factors have on lifespan is as yet unclear.

Squaring the rectangle

The net result of the changes in demographic patterns is summarized in Figure 4. The changing pattern of survival has been described by Fries and Crapo (1981) as 'squaring the rectangle'. Longevity has not increased but the majority of individuals can now expect to live close to their biological maximum. The near logarithmic decline in numbers seen in the mortality data for 1851 is a reflection of environmental factors influencing lifespan rather than genetic factors as seen in the data for 1978.

THE BIOLOGY OF AGEING

Ageing of germ cells

Ageing is a feature primarily of multicellular organisms that depend upon sexual reproduction to continue the species. Single cell organisms show few changes that can be attributed to ageing and many plant species can be

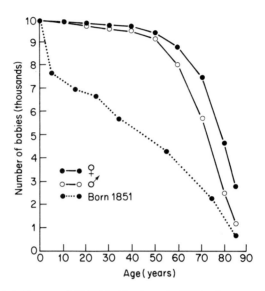

Figure 4. Predicted lifespan of 10 000 babies born in 1978 using mortality data collected 1973–1975. From Carter (1980).

propagated indefinitely by vegetative means. It is essential, however, for the maintenance of a species that the germ cells remain immune to ageing; old organisms that reproduce need to produce healthy offspring. There are many recorded cases of octogenarian and nonagenarian men fathering normal children, indicating that some correctly-functioning sperm are being produced. The numbers of abnormal forms increase with age but these abnormalities are not universal and seem likely to result from extrinsic, environmental effects on the testes. Similarly, women approaching the menopause with 50-year-old ova can produce normal offspring. The increased incidence of genetically abnormal forms again probably results from environmentally damaging factors such as radiation and toxins.

Man is exceptional in having a menopause. Only some inbred forms of mice exhibit similar changes. While most animals show a decline in reproductive capability in ageing there is usually some functioning ovarian tissue containing gametes at the time of death. It is possible that man has evolved the menopause to limit the effects of harmful environmental factors on subsequent generations, although with current knowledge it is hard to see how such evolutionary pressure could have been exerted.

The link between growth and reproduction is of considerable interest. The primary function of all organisms is to reproduce, but in an environment with limited resources there may be insufficient energy supplied to cope with growth and reproduction simultaneously and it is probably therefore advantageous for growth to be completed before reproduction takes place, to prevent competition for resources. In the plant world growth continues throughout life and therefore this division of function cannot occur, but it has been noted that oak trees grow less in years of high seed output (Calow, 1979). Water-boatmen subjected to environmental stress such as nutritional deficiency suffer greater mortality if they are pregnant, because resources are diverted from flight muscle to the eggs (Calow, 1979). Thus growth and subsequent life expectancy are sacrificed for reproduction. Whether such factors are of importance in man remains to be determined.

AGE CHANGES AND DIFFERENCES

Cross-sectional studies tell the observer of differences between the population he is studying. For example, if groups of individuals of different ages are assessed for hearing loss a decline in sensitivity to high frequency sound would be found in the elderly. It would not however be possible to conclude from such a study that the differences found were a result of age change rather than cohort effects. It is conceivable that changes in the pattern of nutrition, noise exposure, drug therapy or many other factors may have had specific effects on populations at particular times in history. Only by performing longitudinal studies can true age changes be demonstrated. Longitudinal studies are expensive, time-consuming and may require extreme altruism on the part of the researcher who may not live to see the results published.

Body constituents

Complex multicellular organisms contain many different types of cells and non-cellular material. It would be unreasonable to suppose that ageing affects all equally. In attempting to classify tissues, the most obvious difference is between those cells that are constantly dividing, those cells which do not divide and remain fixed from birth till death, and the non-cellular material.

Dividing cells

An erythrocyte survives approximately 120 days. During a life of 70 years an individual will therefore have at least 200 complete generations of erythrocytes. Over the 120-day period the cells undergo certain changes which may be classified as age changes but will have no impact on overall age change of the organism. Ageing of the stem cell may produce changes in young erythrocytes in an old organism but in fact relatively little difference is found comparing young cells from a young organism with young cells from an old organism. This holds true for most dividing cells studied and includes leucocytes, gut epithelial cells, epidermal cells and spermatozoa.

Cells that are constantly renewing themselves are also better able to withstand environmental damage so long as the damage does not also involve the stem cell. The skin is able to repair itself after injury; gastritis due to toxins such as alcohol will quickly resolve with abstinence.

Fixed cells

Neurones, myocardial cells, renal parenchymal cells, hepatocytes and ova are all cells which do not replicate. Cell death within an organ will therefore lead to an irreversible decline in function as can be seen in the gradual loss of glomeruli in the kidney leading to a progressive decline in renal function with age. The pigment epithelial cells in the retina responsible for phago-cytosing 250 000 light sensitive membranes daily extruded by the rods and cones are captive macrophages which, with the passage of time, become packed full of waste debris. The cells attempt to extrude the debris through Bruchs membrane producing white plaques visible through the ophthalmo-scope called drusen (after the shiny debris seen at the top of volcanoes). This ageing process sometimes results in clinically significant macular degener-ation. Thus fixed cells are more susceptible to damage through accumulation of waste products, and are less capable of withstanding environmental stress than dividing cells.

Non-cellular material

The effect of age on collagen has been well documented. Increased cross-linkage between collagen fibres leads to a decline in distensibility which can be most easily seen in the dermis, where in combination with fewer elastin fibres there is the classic loss of skin elasticity typical of old age. The increase in cross-links in bone collagen is in part the cause of brittle bones in old age and in the lung again in combination with less elastin there is reduced elastic recoil of the lungs after expansion. The lens of the eye progressively thickens with age as new lens fibres are laid down on top of the old fibres. The lens becomes more rigid, the central portion becomes less accessible to nutrients and soluble proteins precipitate producing cataracts, so called because they are said to produce vision similar to that of looking through a waterfall. Thus changes within non-cellular material play an important role in many of the disorders associated with ageing.

CRITERIA OF AGEING

One of the important advances in medicine over the last forty years has been the realization that disease can be treated in old age. An essential step in this development was the recognition of the differences between normal ageing and disease. The apocryphal story of the elderly man presenting to his doctor with a painful knee illustrates this. Given the explanation that the pain was due to his age the patient accepted it but questioned why his other knee was not also painful as it was of the same age.

Strehler (1962) gave four criteria that he felt needed to be fulfilled before a change could be accepted as due to ageing. The criteria provide a useful framework on which ageing research can be based.

1. Universal

Any change attributed to ageing should develop to a greater or lesser extent in all members of the species. For example to prove that baldness is an ageing phenomena it must be shown that all subjects lose some portion of the hair follicles that they have at maturity.

2. Intrinsic

The changes that are observed should be restricted to those which are of endogenous origin and not the result of extrinsic factors. Thus many of the changes found with ageing in the skin may be seen in an accelerated form in subjects exposed to high doses of ultraviolet radiation. The term photoaging has been given to this phenomenon but it cannot be regarded as a true age change, being the result of exogenous factors. Atheroma is an almost universal finding in the aged in Western society but there is strong evidence that this is diet related and therefore cannot again be regarded as an age change. There may however be underlying ageing factors within the blood vessels which predispose to the deposition of lipids within the wall.

3. Progressive

All true ageing phenomena develop progressively and for this reason it is necessary to distinguish between those effects which have a higher incidence above a certain age but which develop rapidly, and those which progressively develop with increasing age. For example the sudden occlusion of a cerebral artery leading to stroke cannot be regarded as an ageing phenomenon, but as explained above some of the factors leading to the underlying atheroma may result from an age change.

4. Deleterious

This is the most controversial of the criteria. For a change to be regarded as an ageing phenomenon it should be harmful for the organism. If the definition of ageing is limited to the changes occuring after maturity then the criterion is valid. Some of the observed changes are however simply progression of changes which were beneficial to the organism during the period of growth and development. The increased cross-linkage of collagen in bone is important for providing strength during growth. When the same process continues after maturity it ultimately leads to brittle bones. The point at which advantage becomes disadvantage is therefore difficult to ascertain.

The criteria thus provide a strict set of guidelines for classifying ageing phenomena. They are often extremely difficult to prove. If cancer which increases in frequency with age results from an inefficient ageing immune system, is the cancer an age change? If painful knees secondary to osteoarthritis result in impaired mobility, difficulty in shopping and resulting nutritional deficiency, is the malnutrition an ageing phenomenon? Hall (1984) draws the analogy of the multiple layers of an onion, with successive intrinsic and extrinsic factors all interrelating to produce pathology. It is certainly often difficult to separate pathology from physiology in old age.

EXPERIMENTS ON AGEING

For centuries man has attempted to find the elixir of life with little success. More people are achieving an age close to maximum longevity, squaring the survival curve (Fries and Crapo, 1981), but the curve has not yet been shifted to the right. Experiments manipulating the environment have however yielded interesting results worthy of further study.

Nutrition

McCay et al (1935) demonstrated that severe calorie restriction, but with a balanced diet overall, led to an increased longevity in rats compared to those animals fed *ad libitum*. Miller and Payne (1968) showed that the longest lifespan was obtained by supporting maximum growth for the first 120 days followed by a diet just sufficient to maintain weight thereafter. It is suggested that the benefits of dietary restriction may be obtained by a more selective means. Reducing the intake of tryptophan alone depresses physical and reproductive development and may itself increase longevity (Segall and Timiras, 1976).

Dietary restriction early in life in mice appears to improve immune function assessed by lymphocyte responsiveness to mitogens late in life when compared to matched controls and provides a possible explanation for the increased survival (Walford et al, 1973). Andres (1981) reviewed studies on the effect of nutrition on ageing in man. The conclusion was that the heaviest and thinnest cohorts had the shortest survival with the maximum lifespan associated with a weight slightly over the conventionally accepted ideal body weight. The populations identified around the world as possibly containing a high proportion of long-lived individuals all consume fewer calories on average than people in Western society.

Exercise

It is fashionable to believe that exercise is 'good for you'. Experimentally, rats exercised on treadmills live longer (Retzlaff et al, 1966) than controls, and a study on the longevity of endurance skiers in Finland (Karvonen et al, 1974), chosen as a group because of their tendency to continue to ski as a hobby after giving up competition, also have a higher life expectancy than the Finnish population as a whole. The results could however just reflect the effect of covert calorie restriction. Clearly such studies have major methodological problems and we await further evidence before putting on our skis or getting on a treadmill!

Antioxidants

One of the popular theories of ageing suggests that free radical reactions play an important role. Antioxidants should prevent the development of free radicals and if the theory is correct delay the progress of ageing. Ethoxyquin and vitamin E are two antioxidants that have been used experimentally in animal studies with apparent benefit on longevity. Comfort et al (1971) reported prolonged life in C3H mice treated with ethoxyquin but there was also associated weight loss suggesting an effect on calorie intake which itself may have caused the improvement in survival. Miquel et al (1973) showed improved survival in Drosophila treated with vitamin E but this has not been confirmed in other species; indeed in man high doses of vitamin E appears to increase mortality (Enstrom and Pauling, 1982).

Overcrowding

City dwellers are less likely to live to old age than those from rural communities. For the 25 largest cities in the UK, 4.4% of the population reach the age of 75 compared to 8.3% for the population as a whole (Hall, 1984). Whether this observation is related directly to population density or other factors is unclear.

Financial status

The Black report 'Inequalities in Health' (Townsend and Davidson, 1982) highlighted the differences in lifespan between social classes. Unskilled manual workers and skilled manual workers die earlier than those in social classes I and II. Illsley and Le Grand (1987) point out that using the Registrar General's classification of class limits analysis to males between 15 and 64 years and therefore may introduce unacceptable bias. Their preliminary results using a wider analysis of social class suggest that the gap in health status between the rich and poor may be narrowing.

Temperature

It has been demonstrated in several poikilothermic organisms that lowered body temperature results in increased longevity. Liu and Walford (1975), experimenting on fish, transferred mature animals from warm to cold environments and vice versa confirming the advantage of cold to survival. It is difficult to extrapolate these findings to warm blooded animals.

HUMAN LONG-LIVED POPULATIONS

Three remote communities have received considerable scientific attention in recent years because of claims that their populations live to extreme old age: The district of Abkhazia in the Caucasus Mountains of the USSR, the Hunza province in the Karakoram Mountains of northwestern Pakistan, and the village of Vilcabama in the Andes of Ecuador. In a well argued chapter entitled 'The Myth of Methuselah', Fries and Crapo (1981) throw serious doubt on the validity of such claims. Documentation in such isolated communities is usually poor with no registration of births, the strange preponderance of men amongst the centenarians where in all other populations the survivors tend to be women, and the high proportion of married couples both surviving to great old age, defying the laws of probability.

If however such claims are true then the evidence described in previous sections provides some possible explanations because the diets are low in calories and animal fats, physical fitness remains high with people continuing to labour in the fields until death, and overcrowding and the resultant pressures and stresses of industrial life are absent.

THEORIES OF AGEING

There are nearly as many theories of ageing as there are researchers and there may be elements of truth in all of them. It seems unlikely at present that a single explanation will ever be sufficient to explain all the features of ageing.

Wear and tear

An old theory first proposed by Weisman (1882) which states that 'death takes place because a worn out tissue cannot forever renew itself'. Elephants often die because their teeth wear out and they are no longer able to feed adequately. The loss of cartilage from joints in osteoarthritis, while sometimes accelerated by exogenous factors, may be a form of wear and tear ageing. It is however difficult to use this theory more widely to explain other features of ageing.

Accumulation theories

It is suggested that accumulation of waste products within cells leads to a gradual decline in function and ultimately to cell death. Lipofuscin or age pigment accumulates in the cytoplasm of the cells of many tissues, particularly neurones and cardiac muscle. There is a close correlation between the quantity of lipofuscin and the age of the subject. Lipofuscin is formed from a free radical reaction between lipids and protein, and ever since its presence was first observed by Stubel (1911) attempts have been made to attribute declining cell function to it. There is as yet, however, no evidence that the presence of lipofuscin is detrimental to the cell.

The pigment epithelial cells in the retina have already been discussed, but again the accumulation of the waste products from phagocytosis of light-sensitive membranes leading to the changes of macular degeneration could be included in this category of age changes.

Cross-linking

Björksten (1974) was the first to propose that increasing cross-links between macromolecules such as proteins and nucleic acids could lead to them becoming less metabolically active, with the resultant decline in cell function. Verzar (1968) produced evidence to support the hypothesis by demonstrating progressive increases in cross-linkage between collagen fibres in rats tails. Many other workers have confirmed these findings in many of the tissues of the body. An interesting observation is that treating collagen with aldehydes increases the numbers of cross-links. Malondialdehyde is a degradation product of lipid peroxidation suggesting a link with free radical reactions.

Free radical theory

The free radical theory suggests that peroxidation of cellular constituents generates a chain of free radical reactions which cause cumulative damage to cellular components (Harman, 1956). Free radicals are highly unstable molecules lacking one of a pair of electrons which biochemically are constantly attempting to attain stability by withdrawing an electron from a hitherto stable molecule. The reactions tend to result in the formation of inactive polymers of protein, polyunsaturated fatty acids, nucleic acids or combinations of each which may be harmful to the cell. This has however not yet been clearly demonstrated. The theory has led to the trials of anti-oxidants described earlier.

Immunological theories of ageing

The observation that infection, malignancy and autoimmune disease all increase in frequency with age, have led to suggestions that immune failure may play a significant role in ageing of the organism (Walford, 1969). The changes described in the immune system with age are subtle and are not universal. It is difficult to know which comes first, ageing or ageing immunity.

IS AGEING PROGRAMMED OR THE RESULT OF RANDOM ERRORS?

Longevity is species-specific

Each animal species has a fixed maximum lifespan; the mayfly lives 24 hours, the mouse 3 years and man 120 years. Longevity would thus appear to be genetically predetermined.

Effect of parental age

Pearl and Pearl (1934) performed a large longitudinal study of longevity in man and found a positive correlation between a subjects age at death and a 'total index of ancestral longevity' calculated by adding the age at death of the two parents and four grandparents and dividing by six.

Abbott et al (1974) also found that familial longevity had a role to play in determining the longevity of the children but the influence was not as great as that suggested in the earlier study, possibly one year added for every ten years of parental survival.

Twin studies

Kallman and Sander (1949) studied 58 twin pairs to assess the degree of concordance of lifespan. Monozygous twins had mean differences in life-span of 36.9 months. Dizygous twins of the same sex had a mean difference of 78.3 months and dizygous twins of the opposite sex 126.6 months. The differences were statistically significant and would again support the hypothesis that there is a genetic influence on lifespan.

The Hayflick phenomenon

The evidence that cells have a fixed programme determining senescence is strongly supported by the research of Hayflick (1965) on human fibroblasts. Fetal cells cultured in vitro multiplied through 40 cell cycles and then the culture died off. Cells taken from older subjects died in a proportionately shorter time. The number of potential divisions was related to the maximum lifespan of the species being studied. These findings have been criticized as perhaps reflecting inadequate cell culture conditions with lack of nutrients or viral infection, but they have been reproduced by other workers and are worthy of study. Forty cell doublings is however far more than would normally be required during a normal human lifespan and so, even if the experiment is giving true results, its relevance to normal ageing is questionable.

HOW MANY GENES ARE INVOLVED IN AGEING

The evidence available suggests there are only few genes responsible for determining longevity.

Progeria

If only few genes are involved then it might be expected that occasionally, through chance mutation, syndromes would arise with abnormalities of the ageing process. Progeria (premature old age) and progeria-like syndromes are familial conditions with features similar to ageing but occurring early in life. Mean lifespan is usually dramatically shortened, death occurring from cardiac or cerebrovascular disease; presbyopia, articular cartilage destruction and many of the classical features of ageing skin occur. Epstein et al (1966) have shown a decreased number of cell doublings of fibroblasts from patients with progeria.

Individuals with Downs syndrome (trisomy 21) also show some features which could be attributed to accelerated ageing. Life expectancy is usually short with only 20% surviving beyond 30 years, they often have early vascular disease, diabetes mellitus, osteoporosis, cataracts, hair loss, skin atrophy, lipofuscin deposition and autoimmune disease. Features of Alzheimer's disease are sometimes the most striking clinical problem.

Immortal cells

Cells in culture will normally die after a period of division (Hayflick phenomenon). Infecting cells with viral particles particularly retroviruses may transform the cell line to immortality. Viruses only carry small amounts of genetic material suggesting immortality can be confirmed with few genes.

Evolution and longevity

It is estimated that man separated from its common ancestor with the chimpanzee 15 million years ago, a relatively short time in evolutionary terms, and yet the longevity of the two species differs by a factor of more than two, the chimpanzees maximum lifespan being only 45 years (Cutler, 1978). The protein makeup of the chimpanzee and of man are estimated to be 99% similar. Thus a small change in genetic material has resulted in a large change in longevity.

RANDOM ERROR THEORY

The obverse of a genetically determined biological clock mechanism for senescence is the random error hypothesis of Orgel (1963, 1970). Through random errors in DNA replication and RNA transcription faulty proteins would be synthesized leading to a decline in cell function. Protein formation involves a series of complex reactions. Errors in DNA and RNA synthesis are frequent but the cell has repair mechanisms designed for such a situation. An endonuclease breaks the nucleic acid at the abnormal part and a polymerase catalyses the insertion of the correct components. When the repair mechanism fails, aberrant protein synthesis results. This may not lead to significant loss of cellular efficiency but accumulation of errors will ultimately result in cell death, a situation termed 'error catastrophe'. If the aberrant proteins themselves are part of the cell repair mechanism then through a positive feedback loop it would be expected that much more rapid cell death would result.

If the hypothesis is correct it would be expected that senescence would be accompanied by increasing amounts of aberrant protein accumulating in cells and that by causing experimentally the production of abnormal proteins it would be possible to mimic the normal ageing process. The evidence from studies examining these predictions is conflicting but on balance there is more in favour than against. The efficiency of cellular repair mechanisms has been shown in some studies, but not all, to be closely correlated to longevity. One such study is illustrated in Figure 5, where

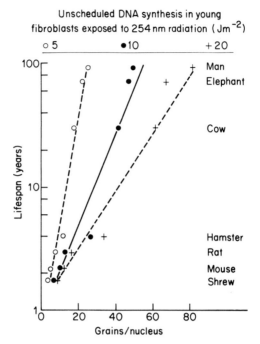

Figure 5. A correlation between the amount of unscheduled DNA synthesis measured 13 hours after exposure to several UV fluences and the estimated lifespan of the species. From Hart and Setlow (1974).

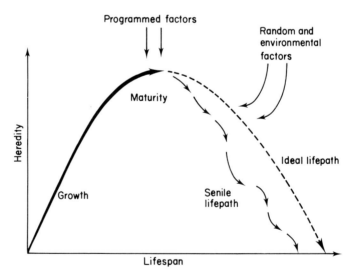

Figure 6. The comparison of lifespan modulation by internal and external factors to the flight path of a projectile, demonstrating the composite effects of programmed and random ageing processes. From Hall (1984).

DNA in fibroblasts was damaged and the efficiency of ultraviolet light excision repair measured.

INTEGRATION THEORIES

Hall (1984) has suggested a way in which programmed and random error theories can be united to provide a coherent picture of ageing. This is illustrated in Figure 6.

Using the analogy of throwing a projectile into the air, the factors which influence the height it reaches and the distance it travels can be compared to the factors determining growth, development and ageing. Genetic factors are equated with the force with which the projectile is initially thrown, controlling differentiation growth and some ageing factors. Under ideal conditions all members of a species will travel the same ideal pathway and have the same lifespan. Random errors and adverse environmental factors however may cause the organism to deviate from the ideal lifepath and result in a shortened lifespan. Thus genetic factors determine interspecies difference in longevity and the environment and random errors determine differences between individuals of species.

SUMMARY

The absolute numbers and proportion of elderly people within society is increasing and will continue to increase into the next century. An understanding of normal biology, physiology and anatomy of ageing are an essential prerequisite for the treatment of pathology in the elderly. Gerontology is a young scientific discipline where important developments are being made. Progress in increasing longevity has so far been limited, but continuing improvements in the quality of life for the elderly remain an attainable goal.

REFERENCES

Abbott MH, Murphy EA, Boling DR (1974) The Familial components in longevity. A study of offspring in nonagenarians II Preliminary analysis of the completed study. *John Hopkins Medical Journal* **134**: 1–16.

Andres R (1981) Aging, diabetes and obesity: standards of normality. *Mount Sinai Journal of Medicine* **48**: 489–495.

Bellamy, D (1985) Biology of Ageing. In Pathy MSJ (ed.) *Principle and Practice of Geriatric Medicine*, pp 67–104. Chichester: John Wiley and Sons.

Björksten J (1974) Cross-linkage and the aging process In Rockstein M (ed.) *Theoretical Aspects of Aging*, p 43. New York: Academic Press.

Butler RN (1979) *The Graying of Nations: Creative responses*. London: Age Concern.

Calow P (1979) The cost of reproduction—A physiological approach *Biological Reviews* **54**: 23–40.

Carter ND (ed.) (1980) *Development, Growth and Ageing*, p 169. London: Croom and Helm.

Comfort A, Youhotsky-Gore I, Pathmanathan K (1971) Effect of ethoxyquin on the longevity of C3H mice. *Nature* **229**: 254–255.

Cutler RG (1978) Evolutionary biology of senescence. In Behnke JA, Finch CE & Moment GD (eds). *The Biology of Aging*. New York: Plenum Press.

Enstrom, JE & Pauling L (1982) Mortality among health-conscious elderly Californians. *Proceedings of the National Academy of Sciences USA*. **79**: 6023-6027.

Epstein CJ, Martin GM, Schultz AL & Motulsky A (1966) Werner's Syndrome *Medicine* **45**: 177–221.

Fries JF & Crapo LM (1981) *Vitality and Aging: implications of the rectangular curve*, p 172. San Franciso: W.H. Freeman.

Gompertz B (1825) On the nature of the function expressive of the law of human mortality and on a new mode of determining life contingencies. *Philosophical Transactions of the Royal Society of London* **11**: 513–585.

Hall DA (1984) *The Biomedical Basis of Gerontology*, pp 18–52. Bristol: J. Wright & Sons.

Hamilton JB & Mestler GE (1969) Mortality and survival: comparison of eunuchs with intact men and women in a mentally retarded population. *Journal of Gerontology* **24**: 395–411.

Harman D (1956) Aging: a theory based on free radical and radiation chemistry. *Journal of Gerontology* **11**: 298–300.

Hart RW & Setlow RB (1974) DNA repair and life span of mammals. In Hanawalt PC & Setlow RB (eds). *Molecular Mechanisms for Repair of DNA*, part B, pp 801–804. New York: Plenum Press.

Hayflick L (1965) The limited in-vitro lifetime of human diploid strains. *Experimental Cell Research* **37**: 614–636.

Illsley R & Le Grand J (1987) *The measurement of inequality in health*. Suntom—Toyoto International Centre for Economics and Related Disciplines, Discussion Paper 12, 30 pp.

Kallman FJ & Sander G (1949) Twin studies on ageing and longevity. *Journal of Heredity* **39**: 349–357.

Karvonen MJ, Klemola H, Virkagarvi, J & Kekkonen A (1974) Longevity of endurance skiers. *Medicine and Science in Sports* **6**: 49–51.

Liu RK & Walford RL (1975) Mid-life temperature transfer effects on life-span of annual fish. *Journal of Gerontology* **30**: 129–131.

McCay CM, Cromwell MF & Maynard LA (1935) The effect of retarded growth upon the length of life span and upon the ultimate body age. *Journal of Nutrition* **10**: 63–79.

Miller DS & Payne PR (1968) Longevity and protein intake. *Experimental Gerontology* **3**: 231–234.

Miquel J, Binnard R & Howard WH (1973) Effects of D.L.-alpha-tocopheral on the lifespan of Drosophila melanogaster. *Gerontologist* **3**: 37–45.

Orgel LE (1963) The maintenance of accuracy of protein synthesis and its relevance to aging. *Proceedings of the National Academy of Sciences USA* **49**: 517–521.

Orgel LE (1970) The maintenance of the accuracy of protein synthesis and its relevance to aging: a correction. *Proceedings of the National Academy of Sciences USA* **67**: 1476.

Pearl R & Pearl RD (1934) *The Ancestry of the Long Lived*. Baltimore: John Hopkins University Press.

Retzlaff E. Fontaine J & Furuta W (1966) Effect of daily exercise on lifespan of albino rats. *Geriatrics* **21**: 171–177.

Rockstein M & Lieberman HM (1958) Survival curves for male and female house-flies (Musca domestica. L.) *Nature* **181**: 787–788.

Segall PE & Timiras PS (1976) Pathophysiologic findings after chronic tryptophane deficiency in rats. *Mechanisms of Ageing and Development* **5**: 109–124.

Strehler BL (1962) *Time, cells and aging*, p 456. New York: Academic Press.

Stubel H (1911) Fluorescenz terscher Geweve in ultraviolettem licht *Pflügers Archive für die gesante Physiologie des Menschen und der Tiere* **142**: 1.

Thompson J (1987) Ageing of the population: contemporary trends and issues *Population Trends* (HMSO) **50**: 18–22.

Townsend P & Davidson N (1982) *Inequalities in Health: The Black Report*, p. 240. London: Penguin.

Verzar F (1968) *Lectures on Experimental Gerontology* Springfield: Thomas.

Walford RL (1969) *The Immunologic theory of Aging*. Copenhagen: Munksgaard.

Walford RL, Liu RK, Gerbase-Delima M, Mathies M & Smith G (1973) Long-term dietary restriction and immune function in mice: response to sheep red blood cells and mitogenic agents. *Mechanism of Ageing and Development* **2**: 447–454.
Weisman A (1882) *Uberdie des lebens* (Concerning Lifespan). Jena: Fisher.

2

Age-related genito-urinary changes

DAVID WARRELL

The changes in the genito-urinary organs of women with advancing age are a consequence not just of the ageing process but also of earlier events, chiefly parturition and the menopause. The tissue changes produced by the combination of these processes often adversely affect the structure and function of the genito-urinary organs.

The aetiology of uterine prolapse provides an example of this interaction. In young nulliparous women in the erect position the axis of the vagina is approximately parallel to the ground. The uterus is positioned over the levator plate by its fascial supports so that the pelvic floor provides support against increases in abdominal pressure and gravitational force. Parturition damages the nerve supply of the striated muscle of the pelvic floor (Allan et al, 1988) and the denervation process continues with ageing. As the pelvic floor weakens it sags and the axis of the vagina approaches the vertical. The uterus is no longer positioned over the levator plate and supported by it so greater strain is put on its fascial supports. This change often takes place at a time when the endopelvic fascia is becoming weaker, for collagen is an important constituent of these supports and is adversely affected both by the menopause and by ageing. In some women the combination of parturition damage, menopausal and ageing tissue changes is so great as to result in uterine prolapse.

The common time to present with uterine prolapse is from middle age onwards, but a dominance of one factor causing damage accounts for the appearance of uterine prolapse at other ages. Gross parturition damage, for example, may cause an early onset. Infrequently uterine prolapse is seen in elderly nulliparous women, when the menopause and ageing have produced sufficient change so as to allow the uterus to prolapse. It is likely such women have an intrinsic fascial weakness for often other members of the family are affected.

HORMONAL CHANGE

In the reproductive years the ovary has three compartments for steroid biosynthesis. These are maturing follicles, corpora lutea and the stroma. At the menopause the remaining primordial follicles which are usually but not always present, cease to respond even to considerable increase in pituitary gonadotrophin levels and the stroma remains as the only source of oestrogen production in the post-menopausal ovary (Mattingly and Huang, 1969). The high concentrations of follicle stimulating hormone (FSH) and luteinizing hormone (LH) found after the menopause are due to the loss of feedback inhibition normally exerted by oestradiol. These levels remain high until old age. The increase in pituitary gonadotrophins is not seen as an acute rise at the cessation of menses but is part of a more gradual change in hypothalmic–pituitary ovarian relationships seen throughout the climacteric.

The changes in ovarian function seen at the climacteric cause a fairly rapid change in the hormone dependent genito-urinary tracts; thereafter the changes are due to ageing and take place more gradually. The waning of ovarian function which results in the menopause is a slow process and may well spread out over 5 or 10 years. However the changes in the genito-urinary tracts consequent on decreased steroid production are only seen at the end of this period when ovulation ceases and oestrogen levels decline to the post-menopausal range.

A minority of women are spared the most marked effects for they convert androstenedione produced in the ovary and adrenal gland into oestrone by aromatization in peripheral fat. To a lesser extent testosterone is converted into oestradiol. In post-menopausal women, plasma levels of oestrone and to a lesser extent oestradiol correlate with body weight and excess body fat (Judd et al, 1976). So it could be anticipated that the hormone-dependent changes would be less evident in well-fleshed women than in thin women. However oestrone which is the predominant hormone has only about one tenth of the biological activity of oestradiol. It seems likely that oestradiol is more important than oestrone in maintaining the state of hormone-dependent tissues in post-menopausal women (Morse et al, 1979). In clinical practice there is no obvious relationship between body build and vaginal oestrogenization.

MACROSCOPIC AND MICROSCOPIC GENITAL TRACT CHANGES

Ovary

The post-menopausal ovary is small, white and wrinkled. As follicular activity ceases there is a continuing involution of the cortex with a relative increase in the medulla. Germinal inclusion cysts are commonly found in the post-menopausal ovary and seem to increase in frequency with age. Lipid droplets can been seen in the stroma suggesting continuing steroidogenesis.

Uterus

When menstruation ceases the uterus and cervix become smaller. This decrease in size is greater in the body of the uterus than in the cervix. The myometrium decreases in bulk, mainly because of a decrease in cell cytoplasm with a consequent appearance of increased nuclear density. Uterine fibroids undergo a similar change. The changes in the endometrium reflect the rate of decline of oestrogen production: the endometrium becomes thin and the distinction between the basal and functional layers is lost; the glands become inactive and mitotic activity ceases. Sometimes these changes take place quite quickly, but it is quite common to see some degree of proliferation and mitotic activity for a year or two after cessation of menstruation. In a high proportion of women the endometrial glands become cystically dilated. This is thought to be due to blockage and is not the end stage of cystic hyperplasia. Mitotic activity ceases and its presence in an established post-menopausal endometrium strongly suggests the administration of exogenous oestrogen or an endogenous source. Total squamous metaplasia occurs in a small number of women (the aetiology of this is not known).

Cervix and vagina

The vaginal fornices become shallow so that the cervix appears nearly flush to the vaginal vault. The vaginal walls depend for immediate support on the so called perivaginal fascia. This is not true fascia but is a sheath composed of smooth muscle, blood vessels, collagen and elastic tissue. After the menopause this layer of tissue becomes thinner. It is logical to accept that low oestrogen levels will reduce the collagen content however the effect of the menopause on the other constituents of this tissue has not been documented. There is considerable change in the perivaginal tissue for the vagina shrinks in length and calibre and becomes less distensible. If the supporting tissue of the vagina has been damaged by childbirth, the further changes consequent on the menopause may lead to vaginal-wall prolapse.

The depth and maturity of the squamous epithelium of vagina and cervix is dependent on adequate levels of circulating oestrogen. After the menopause it becomes thinner and maturation is arrested at the mid zone. There is considerable variation, however, and up to 40% of women retain oestrogenized smears for many years after the menopause (McLennan and McLennan, 1971). The squamo-columnar junction of the cervix frequently recedes into the endocervical canal. The important implication of this is that the area most likely to undergo neoplasia tends to retreat out of reach of the cervical smear spatula, so when taking a smear from a post-menopausal woman it is important to sample the endocervical canal. Since the latter is likely to be narrow the spatula may have to be reshaped in order to enter the canal and obtain an adequate sample of cells.

The atrophy of the vaginal epithelium affects the intracellular production of glycogen, the population of lactobacilli falls and the production of lactic acid diminishes resulting in a shift of the vaginal pH towards alkalinity. This change in pH allows colonization by bacterial pathogens which together with the thinning of the vaginal epithelium account for the common occurrence of bacterial vaginal infection, the so-called atrophic vaginitis. The combination of atrophic epithelial changes, frequent infection and reduced vaginal volume account for the symptoms of vaginal discomfort and pain on coitus so often experienced by post-menopausal women.

Vulva

In post-menopausal women the vulva shrinks and the epidermis thins, although there may be increased keratinization. These post-menopausal changes often coincide with the appearance of a vulval dystrophy—a common and underdiagnosed condition. Thus vulval skin irritation and discomfort are common symptoms in post-menopausal women.

Bladder and urethra

Three major factors deleteriously influence urinary function as a woman passes through the menopause and grows old. First of all the urothelium of the bladder and urethra becomes thinner and infection more common both giving an increased trigger to micturition; secondly the pelvic floor and the urethral sphincter become weaker, rendering the woman more likely to develop prolapse and stress incontinence; thirdly ageing causes deterioration of neurological control of bladder function and both impairment of inhibition and voiding problems are common.

The urothelium of the bladder changes with age. Jacob et al (1978), in an electron microscopy study of normal bladder epithelium from patients age 60 upwards, report areas of undifferentiated cells only two cells deep scattered among normal bladder transitional epithelium which is three to four layers deep. The urothelium of the urethra and trigone is, like the vagina, hormone-dependent although it does not have such a uniform response as the vagina. In clinical practice, a red, tender external urethral meatus is common in old women; this is often erroneously labelled as a urethral caruncle when at biopsy it is found to be only atrophy. Carlile et al (1987) report that in the urethra there is a gradual change from squamous to columnar epithelium with advancing age and that more squamous type epithelium is preserved at the distal end of the urethra. This observation accords with the finding of oestrogen receptors in the lower urinary tract (Iosif et al, 1981).

No changes in detrusor mass have been reported either in humans or animals; however, all studies of symptomatic elderly women have shown a considerable incidence of trabeculation, i.e. evidence of neurological disease. In the urethra there is a relative decrease in the volume of striated muscle and blood vessels and an increase in the relative volume of connective tissue. There seems to be no change in urethral smooth muscle with age (Carlile et al, 1981). Intrinsic urethral occlusive forces become weaker with age (Raz and Kaufman, 1977).

Changes in urinary control

The neurological control of micturition is complicated. (The subject has been reviewed in detail by Torrens and Morrison, 1987.) In essence the effect of higher control is inhibitory and the major effect of ageing and brain failure is to reduce the capacity to inhibit. Impairment in the co-ordination of the bladder and the urethral sphincter during voiding is also common.

Patterns of micturition alter with advancing age. Nocturnal frequency is the commonest symptom affecting two out of three old people (Brocklehurst et al, 1971). Loss of urinary control is common. In middle age the prevalence of troublesome urinary incontinence is probably about 10%. In old age this figure increases: there is considerable variation according to the population studied but it may be as high as 40% over the age of 65 (Milne, 1976).

Ouslander et al (1986) report a detailed study of elderly women with incontinence and contrast the findings in this group with a similar study of continent women. The most common urodynamic findings in the incontinent group were impaired voiding with residual urine, a reduced bladder capacity, an impaired capacity to inhibit and a weak urethral sphincter. All these findings were present in the continent group albeit with reduced incidence. Trabeculation was noted in both groups. These authors make the point that approximately one third of the patients had multiple urodynamic findings emphasizing that several pathologies were often present in one patient. This study is in accord with all previous reports highlighting the importance of abnormalities of bladder function often in association with trabeculation in the aetiology of old age incontinence.

The loss of urinary control commonly found in old age may be due to the untreated presence of a problem which has been present for many years such as a weak sphincter, but it is much more likely to be due to a neurological disorder affecting bladder function. This may be due to a recent central nervous system abnormality such as stroke or dementia. In some women the neurological disorder is not so evident; many of these have other pathology such as atrophic urethritis or prolapse as well. The likely finding of several causes for incontinence in any one patient makes investigation worthwhile, for though the neurological problem may resist treatment, other causes contributing to incontinence, e.g. an atrophic urethritis, can often be satisfactorily treated with substantial improvement in urinary control.

Pelvic floor

The pelvic floor becomes weaker and sags with advancing age. This finding was documented by Berglas and Ruben (1953) using a technique of levator myography in which water soluble contrast material was injected into the muscle of the pelvic floor and the subject X-rayed whilst erect. This unique study showed that the vaginal axis changes from the horizontal towards the vertical with parity and age and is most marked in women with genital tract prolapse. Smith et al (1989) showed that partial denervation of the pelvic floor is found in women with genital tract prolapse and increases with age. The damage to the nerve supply of the pelvic floor and to the anal and urethral striated sphincters occurs at parturition (Allan et al, 1988) and further denervation takes place as an ageing change.

Ageing changes in the endopelvic fascia, i.e. the supports of the pelvic viscera, have not been studied. There is, however, a strong clinical impression of a weakening of these tissues. Collagen is an important part of these supports and its known deterioration after the menopause and in old age provides some rationale for this observation.

Genital tract prolapse

The factors causing this problem (i.e. childbirth damage to endopelvic fascia and to the nerve supply of the pelvic floor together with the weakening of fascial supports consequent on the menopause) commonly summate to produce a clinically evident genital prolapse in middle age. However, elderly women sometimes present with a surprisingly short history of prolapse. There is a clinical impression that there may be damage to the sensory as well as motor nerves because many patients with a large prolapse seem to experience little discomfort. A large cysto-urethrocele is often thought to cause difficulty voiding giving rise to a residual urine and infection. Similarly rectocele is often blamed for an impairment in the capacity to defaecate and constipation. It is common to find abnormalities of bladder or bowel function in association with prolapse. However the clinician should not leap to the conclusion that the prolapse is causing the disturbance of visceral function. Many women live with quite a large cystocele or rectocele without symptoms. Investigation of visceral function of symptomatic patients with prolapse will often reveal another cause for the visceral upset such as an areflexic bladder to account for voiding problems or blunted rectal sensation to account for the symptom of difficult defaecation or constipation.

CONCLUSION

Multiple pathology is a characteristic of geriatric medicine and disturbances of the function of the pelvic viscera in old women are no exception. Nevertheless detailed clinical assessment together with appropriate studies of bladder and rectal function usually reveal the pathologies causing the disturbance. This effort is worthwhile as a diagnostic exercise alone; however in many cases a treatable pathology is found and the patient benefited.

REFERENCES

Allan RE, Hosker GL, Smith ARB & Warrell DW (1988) The role of pregnancy and childbirth in partial denervation of the pelvic floor. *Neurology and Urodynamics* **7:** 237–239.
Berglas B & Rubin IC (1953) Study of the supportive ligaments of the uterus by levator myography surgery. *Gynaecology and Obstetrics* **97:** 677–692.
Brocklehurst JC, Fry J, Griffiths L & Kalton G (1971) Dysuria in old age. *Journal of the American Geriatric Society* **19:** 582–592.
Carlile AE, Davies I, Faragher E, Rigby A & Brocklehurst JC (1987) Age in the human female urethra. *Neurology and Urodynamics* **6:** 149–150.

Iosif CS, Batras EKA & Astred B (1981) Oestrogen receptors in the human female lower urinary tract. *American Journal of Obstetrics and Gynecology* **141:** 817–820.

Jacob J, Ludgate CA, Forde J & Tullock WS (1978) Recent observations on the ultrastructure of human urothelium—normal bladder of elderly subjects. *Cell and Tissue Research* **193:** 543–560.

Judd HL, Lucas WE & Yen SCC (1976) Serum 17 oestradiol and oestrone levels in post menopausal women with and without endometrial cancer. *Journal of Clinical Endocrinology and Metabolism* **43:** 272–278.

Mattingly RF & Huang WY (1969) Steroidogenesis of the menopausal and post menopausal ovary. *American Journal of Obstetrics and Gynecology* **93:** 1102–1111.

McLennan MT & McLennan CE (1971) Oestrogenic status of menstruating and post menopausal patients assessed by cervico-vaginal smears. *Obstetrics and Gynaecology* **37:** 325–330.

Milne JS (1976) In Willington WL (ed.) *Prevalence of incontinence in elderly age groups*, pp 9–21. London: Academic Press.

Morse AR, Hutton JD, Jacob HS, Murray MAF & James VHT (1979) Relation between the karyopyknotic index and plasma oestrogen concentrations after the menopause. *British Journal of Obstetrics and Gynaecology* **86:** 981–983.

Ouslander JG, Hepps K, Raz S & Su HL (1986) Genito urinary dysfunction in a geriatric outpatient population. *Journal of the American Geriatric Society* **34:** 507–514.

Raz S & Kaufman JJ (1977) Carbon dioxide urethral pressure profile in female incontinence. *Journal of Urology* **117:** 765–769.

Smith ARB, Hosker GL & Warrell DW (1989) Partial denervation of the pelvic floor in the aetiology of genital tract prolapse. *Journal of Obstetrics and Gynaecology* **96:** 24–29.

Torrens M & Morrison JFB (1987) *The Physiology of the lower urinary tract*. Berlin: Springer-Verlag.

3

Medical aspects of surgery in the elderly patient

DAVID GWYN SEYMOUR

It is often stated by those dealing with elderly surgical patients that 'age itself should be no bar to surgery' (Seymour and Vaz, 1987). The management of elderly surgical patients presents a number of special problems, however, many of them medical. This is the justification for a review, such as this, which is written from the medical standpoint. At present, patients over 65 make up about a quarter of all surgical admissions in Britain and in some specialties such as urology half the patients are over 65 years of age (Seymour, 1986). While patients over 65 make up only 5–10% of gynaecology admissions, many of the more extensive gynaecological procedures, such as those for pelvic malignancy, are carried out in middle-aged and elderly patients (Jaluvka, 1980). The literature on the elderly gynaecological patient undergoing surgery is, however, small and most of the information in this chapter derives from the much more extensive general surgical and orthopaedic literature.

AGE AND SURGICAL RISK

Coincidental medical diseases

The older a patient is, the more likely is it that one or more coincidental medical diseases are present. In a recent review of general surgical patients aged over 65 in Cardiff (Vaz and Seymour, 1988), only 20% of patients were free of preoperative medical problems and 30% of patients had three or more problems. The latter group had three times the postoperative mortality rate of the former and postoperative cardiovascular and respiratory problems were also significantly increased. Similarly, in patients undergoing surgery on the colon, Boyd et al (1980) and Greenburg et al (1981) showed that it was preoperative disease rather than age which was the main determinant of immediate postoperative outcome. Long-term survival after surgery in the elderly is also closely related to preoperative medical problems (Andersen and Ostberg, 1972). The fact that many postoperative complications have their roots in pre-existing disease is a strong argument for careful preoperative medical assessment in the elderly.

Table 1. Postoperative mortality rates in the elderly.

Reference	Type of surgery	Lowest age	n	Mortality rates (%)			
				Elective	Non-elective	Excluding carcinomatosis	Total
Farrow et al (1982)	All types	65	18860	—	—	—	6.3
Stephen (1986)	All types	70	1000	4.0	20.4	4.8	5.8
Seymour and Pringle (1983)	General	65	258	6.0	27.0	5.8	12.0
Seymour and Vaz (1988)	General	65	288	2.8	12.7	3.8	5.2
Greenburg et al (1985)	Colonic	70	163	7.5	23.3	—	10.4
Reiss et al (1987)	Abdominal	70	1000	9.7	19.7	10.9	13.6
Jaluvka (1980)	Gynaecological	60	6658				5.9 (age 60–64)
							7.8 (age 65–69)
							8.7 (age 70–74)
							8.9 (age 75–79)
							13.8 (age 80+)

Emergency presentation

There is an increased tendency for elderly patients to present non-electively. In the recent Cardiff study, 19% of general surgical patients aged between 65 and 74 were admitted non-electively, but in the over-75 group the non-elective admission rate was 34%. This trend has been noted repeatedly in the past in data relating to the whole of Scotland (Seymour and Pringle, 1982a) and in a large anaesthetic study carried out in the University Hospital of Wales (Fowkes et al, 1982). The reasons why age and non-elective surgery tend to go together are complex. There is some evidence (Fenyo, 1974; Clinch et al, 1984) that elderly people may be less aware of surgical problems such as peptic ulceration until they become so acute as to demand immediate attention. The general feeling among elderly people and their carers that they are 'too old for surgery' might also contribute to late presentation (Seymour, 1986). It has been tentatively estimated that a third of non-elective general surgical admissions in the elderly might have been open to earlier elective surgical intervention. Not all non-elective admissions lead to non-elective surgery and not all non-elective operations are true emergencies. The recent CEPOD report (Buck et al, 1987) recommended that surgical operations be classed as 'emergencies' if no delay at all was possible, and as 'urgent' if a few hours delay was acceptable. Non-elective surgery tends to be associated with rates of mortality in the elderly which are three to four times higher than those found in elective cases (see Table 1). Part of this mortality may be unavoidable as the time for medical preparation of the patient may be short. However, there is also concern that 'out of hours' surgery is performed by less experienced members of the surgical team (Sherlock et al, 1984; Buck et al, 1987).

Atypical presentation

There is a tendency for certain medical and surgical complications to present atypically in some elderly patients. Thus, sepsis may occur with no pyrexia; myocardial infarction may present as dyspnoea or arrhythmia rather than chest pain; fluid–electrolyte imbalance may present as delirium.

Reduction of homeostatic reserve

Age may also affect the ability of a patient to metabolize drugs or deal with the stress of medical and surgical complications. A general feature of ageing is a reduction in homeostatic reserve so that, for instance, the ability to recover from fluid overload or acidosis may be reduced in even apparently fit elderly patients (Seymour and Seymour, 1988). Drug handling also tends to be altered with age which is especially important in the perioperative period where a large number of anaesthetic and other drugs are likely to be offered.

POSTOPERATIVE MORTALITY

Many reviews of surgery in the elderly lay particular emphasis on the increased rate of postoperative mortality associated with advanced age. There is no doubt that elderly patients tend to have higher rates of mortality than younger patients undergoing a similar operation (Greenburg et al, 1981; Fowkes et al, 1982) and the combination of old age and non-elective surgery appears to be particularly dangerous (see Table 1 for recent reviews). The interpretation of data about postoperative mortality, however, is not as straightforward as it might at first seem and there is a very real danger that information such as that contained in Table 1 will be used as an excuse to deny potentially useful surgery to the elderly.

Seymour and Pringle (1982a) have argued that we should distinguish deaths following potentially curative surgery (such as a pulmonary embolus in a patient undergoing a hernia operation) from deaths related to the progression of serious underlying surgical disease (such as carcinomatosis in patients undergoing a palliative operation). More recently, the audit of perioperative deaths carried out by The Association of Anaesthetists and The Association of Surgeons of Great Britain and Ireland (Buck et al, 1987) has stressed the importance of registering whether mortality was due to surgery, anaesthesia, presenting surgical disease, or intercurrent disease. It is to be hoped that all future studies will accept this CEPOD classification. While the CEPOD audit considered all age-groups, 79% of perioperative mortality was in patients aged 65 and over. Depending on whether surgeons or anaesthetists were making the assessment, intercurrent disease was thought to have contributed to death in between 44% and 52% of cases. Progress of the presenting surgical disease was blamed in about two thirds of cases. Anaesthesia on its own was a very rare cause of death, even in the very elderly.

Over the last two decades, a number of studies have looked at the main reasons for postoperative mortality in the elderly. Among the 'medical' causes cardiovascular problems, respiratory complications and pulmonary embolism are the most prominent with pulmonary embolism tending to be particularly high following orthopaedic operations and operations for pelvic malignancy (Palmberg and Hirsjarvi, 1979; Jaluvka, 1980). It is possible, however, that the overall rate of pulmonary embolism has been decreasing over the last decade because of earlier mobilization and more widespread use of prophylaxis. This is considered further below. Of the 'surgical' causes of death following laparotomy, sepsis remains an important problem in general and gynaecological surgery (Jaluvka, 1980). The prophylactic use of antibiotics is also considered below and appears to be an important method of reducing postoperative mortality.

Before leaving the topic of postoperative mortality, a few technical points need to be made. When reading reports it is important to note whether the mortality rate refers to the immediate postoperative period or, as is more usual, to the number of deaths occurring in hospital. The CEPOD report (Buck et al, 1987) examined all deaths occurring within 30 days of an operative procedure, but found that 75% of the deaths had occurred by the fifteenth day. In a series of elderly gynaecological patients (Jaluvka, 1980) the corresponding figure was 80%. In operations for fractured neck of femur it is customary to report the mortality rate not just at one month but at three, six and twelve months in recognition that the mortality rate of fractured femur patients is higher than the age-adjusted average for at least six months after the fracture. When using centrally-collected data (such as the Hospital Activity Analysis in Britain) as the basis for analysis it is important to recognize that errors in coding may be surprisingly common (Rees, 1982; Whates et al, 1982; Buck et al, 1987).

METHODS OF PREOPERATIVE ASSESSMENT

A number of recent reviews have dealt with the general assessment of surgical patients of all ages (Masey and Burton, 1987; Merli and Weitz, 1987; Norman et al, 1988) and there is little point in repeating all this general information here. For this reason, the remainder of this chapter is concerned with aspects of assessment that are particularly relevant to the elderly, dealing with each major system in turn.

Respiratory

Respiratory disease in the general population becomes more prevalent with increasing age up to about the age of 75, although after that there may be a levelling off. One explanation for this is that patients with more severe forms of respiratory disease do not survive into older age (Caird and Akhtar, 1972). The prevalence of preoperative respiratory disease in elderly surgical patients has been examined in three recent studies. Vaz and Seymour (1988) and Seymour and Pringle (1983) looked at general surgical patients over the age of 65 in Cardiff and Dundee respectively, while Stephen (1986) made a retrospective study of patients aged 70 years and over undergoing all types of surgery. Between 28 and 29% of patients in the three studies had symptoms or signs of lung disease; 14 to 21% of patients had chronic bronchitis (as judged by a history of cough and sputum for more than three months of the year, more than two years running) but this history was twice to three times as common in men as in women. This sex difference appeared to be entirely due to different smoking habits in the two sexes.

The estimated postoperative incidence of respiratory problems varies greatly from study to study depending on the definitions used. In the recent Cardiff study of general surgical patients, the overall incidence of respiratory complications was almost 40%, which is in keeping with the earlier study in Dundee. However, 17% of the patients in Cardiff were diagnosed as having simple atelectasis only, and if these are excluded then the postoperative estimates are 10% for pneumonia and 12% for acute bronchitis. Retrospective studies tend to give a much lower incidence of postoperative respiratory problems but it is likely that minor cases are being missed. Thus Stephen (1986) mentions only five non-fatal, acute respiratory problems in 1000 patients and only seven cases of respiratory failure. In addition, he notes that 4% had atelectasis. Other retrospective studies have placed the incidence of postoperative respiratory problems in elderly general surgical patients between 20 and 40% (Noviant et al, 1976; Mlynek et al, 1977;

Garibaldi et al, 1981). The vast majority of respiratory complications are non-fatal but it must be remembered that of all postoperative deaths that occur in elderly general surgical patients between one sixth and one third have respiratory causes (Seymour and Vaz, 1987).

A number of factors have been shown to increase the risk of post-operative respiratory complications in the elderly. The most important are preoperative chest disease, the site of the surgical incision (incisions near the diaphragm are more likely to cause postoperative chest infections) and smoking. These three risk factors together with volume depletion have recently been combined by multiple logistic regression into a predictor which may prove to be clinically useful (Seymour, 1988). Gross obesity and non-elective surgery may also be important factors in some patients (Seymour and Vaz, 1987). In high-risk respiratory cases, formal pulmonary function may be advisable (Gass and Olsen, 1986; Tisi, 1987).

In the last 20 years, great advances have been made in the understanding of the pathophysiology of postoperative respiratory complications. Full accounts of these developments can be found in a number of excellent reviews (Peters, 1979; Tisi, 1979; Bartlett, 1980; Lewis, 1980). The main finding of this recent research has been that the majority of postoperative complications appear to begin with atelectasis. In many patients this resolves but in some cases it becomes complicated to form frank pneumonia. The atelectasis does not appear to be caused by retention of secretions (as was previously thought), but rather seems to be due to collapse of small basal airways of the lung. The closing volume of the lung is that lung volume at which small airway closure begins to occur on expiration and it therefore follows that the higher the closing volume, the more likely is small airways closure and atelectasis. It has been established that age is one of the major factors causing the closing volume to rise (Hedley-Whyte et al, 1976; Cotes, 1979) which probably explains the higher than average rate of atelectasis and respiratory infection in elderly patients.

Another factor contributing to postoperative respiratory complications in patients of all ages, is a reduction in the sustained maximal inspirations (SMIs or sighs) which normally occur 5–10 times an hour. These SMIs can be abolished by over-sedation or pain, and atelectasis is the likely result. Elderly patients tend to be more sensitive to the effects of sedation and their respiratory control mechanisms may also become less precise with age, again making them increasingly liable to postoperative respiratory complications.

This new research work has had important implications in the prevention and treatment of postoperative respiratory complications.The main development is that modern physiotherapy techniques tend to stress inspiration in preference to the 'classical' methods of expiration, promotion of cough, and 'raising the sputum'. A simple device which appears to be effective in encouraging inspiration in young and middle-aged surgical patients is the incentive spirometer. Recent work has tested out the incentive spirometer in an older population, and results on the whole are promising (Castillo and Haas, 1985; Stock et al, 1985). The use of the incentive spirometer and other devices is widespread in the United States (O'Donohue 1985a,b) but tends to be reserved only for particularly high-risk patients in the United Kingdom.

The highest rates of postoperative respiratory complications occur in operations involving thoracotomy or incisions near the diaphragm. From this point of view gynaecology patients tend to be of lower risk. However, smokers and obese patients undergoing abdominal procedures need to be observed with care particularly in the early postoperative period. Even with close observation, the diagnosis of respiratory complications may present difficulties. Geriatricians are well acquainted with elderly patients whose respiratory infections present as drowsiness or confusion rather than pyrexia and productive cough. The peak incidence for chest complications in the elderly is between two and four days postoperatively and in high-risk patients close observation for the first week is advisable.

Cardiovascular

Depending on the definitions used, up to 50% of elderly people have some evidence of preoperative cardiovascular disease (Boyd et al, 1980; Stephen, 1986; Reiss et al, 1987; Seymour, 1988). The two major postoperative complications which occur are myocardial infarction with an incidence of 1–3% and cardiac failure which is found in 5–10% of postoperative elderly general surgical patients (Seymour and Pringle, 1983; Seymour, 1988). Myocardial infarctions are easy to miss in the postoperative period as at least half of them occur without pain (Becker and Underwood, 1987). Most infarctions in the elderly occur in the first three postoperative days and serial ECGs are advisable during this period. The use of cardiac enzymes to diagnose postoperative myocardial infarction can be a problem following surgical trauma, but special isoenzymes appear to be useful in this respect (Loeb et al, 1985).

A number of preoperative risk factors are associated with an increased incidence of postoperative cardiovascular complications in certain groups of elderly surgical patients (Table 2). However, the prediction of cardio-vascular risk in individual patients has proved much more difficult. Myo-cardial infarction has proved particularly difficult to predict. Part of the reason for this difficulty is the relative rareness of this complication, but the major difficulty is probably related to the fact that no non-invasive test gives a detailed picture of the state of the coronary arteries. Attempts to predict coronary vasculature, using preoperative thallium scanning and exercise testing (Boucher et al, 1985; Coriat et al, 1985; Gerson et al, 1985; Morise et al, 1987) have been made but these can only be regarded as experimental to date. Changes on the preoperative electrocardiogram (ECG) give only a rough indication of the state of the coronary arteries and have little predic-tive value (Seymour et al, 1983). Intraoperative myocardial ischaemia is even more difficult to measure but may be important in the aetiology of postoperative infarcts (Slogoff and Keats, 1985; Yousif et al, 1987).

Attempts to predict postoperative cardiac failure have met with a little more success. Earlier work was concerned almost exclusively with cardiac

Table 2. Pre-operative risk factors and postoperative cardiovascular complications in the elderly. From Seymour and Vaz (1987), with permission.

Preoperative risk factor	Postoperative CVS complications—increase in relative risk			
	Myocardial infarction	Cardiac death	All CVS complications	Comments
Age over 70	↑2–4×	↑2–12×	↑2–3×	Age effects much less when patients with known heart disease excluded
Emergency admission		↑4× (in cardiac surgery)	↑2×	
Myocardial infarction within three months	↑5–8×*	↑5–8×*		⎱ Studies included middle-aged and elderly
Myocardial infarction 3–6 months before	↑2–4×*	↑2–4×*		⎰
Stable angina, controlled heart failure		↑1.5–2×	↑2–3×	
Acute heart failure	?↑2×	↑10–15×		
Dyspnoea on moderate exercise	↑2–4×	↑2–4×	↑2–4×	Potentially treatable risk factor
Sex, obesity, smoking, diabetes, systolic blood pressure	No proven correlation with adverse CVS outcome in elderly			

*Relative to old myocardial infarction.

surgery and the majority of patients were middle-aged rather than elderly. In addition, as part of their cardiac 'work-up', direct measurement of left ventricular function was available. Recent research interest has turned to the 'cardiac patient undergoing non-cardiac surgery' and it is possible that, in the future, non-invasive measurements of left ventricular function (such as nuclear cardiology or echocardiography) will be used to predict post-operative cardiac failure in elderly surgical patients. Attempts have also been made to develop multivariate indices which will be able to predict postoperative cardiac complications from readily-available bedside observations. A much-quoted earlier example of such a multivariate index has been that of Goldman et al (1977), but several reports since then (Waters et al, 1981; Jeffrey et al, 1983; Gerson et al, 1985; Becker, 1986) have found this index to have little predictive value in new sets of patients. New predictive indices have been presented by Detsky et al (1986a,b) and Larsen et al (1987) and may prove clinically useful.

What is the message of this research for bedside CVS evaluation of the preoperative elderly patient at present? A history of myocardial infarction in the last three to six months is an accepted risk factor for perioperative infarction and elective surgery should probably be delayed if possible. Frank symptoms of cardiac failure suggest that cardiac reserve is effectively nil and are likely to be associated with a high rate of postoperative failure and cardiac mortality. In such circumstances it is highly advisable to improve cardiac function by medical means prior to surgery and at least two American studies have shown the value of intensive monitoring in such patients using a Swan–Ganz catheter and an intra-arterial line (Babu et al, 1980; Del Guercio and Cohn, 1980). If a patient is taking cardiac drugs such as digoxin or beta-blockers prior to surgery, the usual advice is not to discontinue them (Seymour, 1986) unless they are causing toxicity. Hypertensive patients tend to have cardiovascular instability and are liable to swings of high and low blood pressure during anaesthesia and surgery (Goldman and Caldera, 1979). However, these swings are not necessarily improved by acute treatment of hypertension in newly-diagnosed cases and the recommendation of anaesthetists is often to tolerate moderate degrees of hypertension, say up to a diastolic of 110, provided there is no cardiac decompensation (Prys-Roberts, 1979). Such patients need to be watched particularly carefully in the operative and postoperative period, however. While diabetes is well known to be associated with arterial disease in the population in general, no study to date has linked diabetes as an independent risk factor with postoperative cardiovascular complications.

Neurological

Postoperative stroke is a surprisingly rare occurrence in elderly general surgical patients. It can be expected in about 1% of general surgical patients aged 65 or more (Knapp et al, 1981; Vaz and Seymour, 1988) and is seen in around 3% of postoperative patients over the age of 80 (Corman, 1979). There is anecdotal evidence that a stroke in the two to three months prior to surgery increases the risk postoperatively, but this is difficult to prove statistically because of the low incidence of postoperative stroke. Except in the field of open-heart surgery it has also been surprisingly difficult to link the incidence of preoperative cerebral vascular disease with postoperative stroke (Gardner et al, 1985). In the early days of open-heart surgery, embolic strokes were quite common, but the incidence appears to be falling with better technology. However, close observation following open-heart surgery will still detect focal neurological signs in around 60% of patients (Smith et al, 1986; Shaw et al, 1987).

Postoperative delirium

Lipowski (1980) has described three types of delirium that can occur in the immediate postoperative period. The first of these *emergence delirium* which occurs immediately after waking from anaesthesia and appears to be as common in the young as in the elderly. *Interval delirium* is the type most often encountered on the wards. Its peak incidence is around two to three days postoperatively although it can occur on day one and be delayed as long as ten days. It is much commoner in the elderly than in the young and appears postoperatively in around 10% of patients after the age of 65 (Seymour and Pringle, 1983; Seymour, 1988). *Delirium tremens* is due to alcohol withdrawal and is more commonly seen in young patients, but it must not be forgotten that elderly patients may have significant alcohol intakes and not necessarily report them to their doctors.

The common causes of postoperative delirium in non-cardiac surgery are acute infection, other acute medical diseases, hypoxia, fluid and electrolyte imbalance, sedation, analgesia, anaesthetic drugs, and untreated pain (Lipowski, 1980). The treatment of delirium is primarily that of the underlying condition and our own experience is that about one third of postoperative cases are due to respiratory infection and one fifth are due to cardiac failure. There is usually little problem in recognizing a hyperactive, delirious patient, but 'quiet delirium' can also occur and may be overlooked. The latter type of patient may appear apathetic and undemanding and it is only on more detailed examination that clouding of consciousness (the key feature of delirium according to the American DSM III Classification) is discovered. Sedatives are more often a cause of delirium than a help in its management and may have disastrous effects if the underlying cause of the delirium is hypoxia. In some conditions, however, a degree of sedation is indicated and a small dose of a phenothiazine such as thioridazine is a useful first line of therapy.

Does dementia ever occur as the result of anaesthesia alone?

This is a question of central interest to every elderly patient undergoing surgery, but the results of research are very reassuring. In 1955, Bedford tried to explore a number of cases of patients who had 'never been the same since the operation'. In a retrospective survey over a five-year period in the Oxford area he could identify only 18 elderly patients who had developed an unequivocal dementia directly following surgery. He found that on close questioning, the majority of patients who were claimed to have post-operative dementia had already had signs of dementia prior to the operation. A follow-up study six years later (Simpson et al, 1961) undertook the mammoth task of prospective testing. Again the incidence of postoperative dementia was found to be extremely low and only one case in 678 elderly patients was detected. While a dementia occurring for the first time after surgery thus appears to be rare, transient changes in performance on psycho-motor testing (which are by definition not dementia) are almost universal even in younger patients but are particularly marked in the elderly. The usual pattern is for such tests to be impaired for about three days after major surgery but to return to normal at about a week. The degree of impairment is often subtle and few of these patients exhibit frank delirium.

Nutritional

Under-nutrition

There is a large and growing literature on under-nutrition in surgical patients, although the grossest examples of protein and calorie malnutrition tend to occur in general surgery particularly in patients with malignancy of the gastrointestinal tract. Patients with fractured necks of femur are also a group where under-nutrition appears to be more common (Bastow et al, 1983). Added nutritional problems are likely to occur when the surgery causes a delay in oral nutrition because of bowel preparation before operation, and prolonged ileus afterwards. From the above remarks it will be seen that under-nutrition is likely to be less of a problem to the gynaecological surgeon dealing with the elderly than in the field of general or orthopaedic surgery. For this reason, only a few general concepts are mentioned here, and the interested reader should consult more detailed sources (see references in Seymour, 1986).

It is useful to think of under-nutrition in two categories. The first of these is combined protein and calorie malnutrition. Such patients tend to be under-weight and are usually readily recognizable. The second type of patient has protein malnutrition out of proportion to calorie malnutrition, and may not be as easy to recognize. Serum albumin tends to be depleted in this second group, however, and their extracellular space may be expanded. Immunological impairment is also more common in this second group than in the group with combined protein and calorie malnutrition. Some authors refer to the second group of patients as having 'adult kwashiorkor'.

A variety of anthropometric and biochemical tests have been suggested for preoperative nutritional assessment. Earlier reports tended to stress anthropometric measurements and some of these claimed that 65% of general surgical patients were malnourished, causing Wilcutts (1977) and Gray and Gray (1979) to doubt the relevance of many of the measurements that were being used. Most authors now consider that the true incidence of significant under-nutrition in elderly general surgical patients is much less than 65% and may be as low as 5%. Some authoritative sources (Jeejebhoy and Meguid, 1986; Hill, 1987; Detsky et al, 1987) claim that simple visual inspection is as good as anthropometric measurement for general clinical purposes, but recommend estimation of plasma proteins as a guide to visceral protein depletion.

The use of serum albumin as a nutritional marker has also caused confusion in the literature. While it is true that serum albumin tends to fall with under-nutrition (particularly that of the adult kwashiorkor type), a fall in serum albumin is also seen in acutely ill patients as part of the 'stress' response (Starker et al, 1986; Burns, 1988). This means that patients with a low serum albumin may be protein-depleted, physiologically stressed, acutely ill, chronically ill, or a mixture of all of these. Serum albumin on its own is therefore not a reliable indicator of protein depletion, but it is a useful parameter to measure as a general indicator of 'ill-health'. A serum albumin of 34 g/litre or less has been associated with a significant rise of postoperative complications (particularly those due to sepsis) and mortality in general surgical patients (Seymour, 1986). This correlation with postoperative mortality and morbidity is present even when patients with carcinomatosis (who tend to have a low albumin) are excluded from the analysis.

Obesity

It is likely that the gynaecological surgeon will encounter more obesity than under-nutrition in elderly patients. Obesity can present the operating surgeon with technical problems and this probably explains a rise in incidence of wound complications in the obese (Pasulka et al, 1986; Seymour, 1986). It has been difficult to prove that obesity is linked with postoperative 'medical' complications except in those who are 100% over-weight where respiratory complications are more common (Seymour, 1986).

A recent review of obese patients of all ages (Pasulka et al, 1986) suggests that deep venous thrombosis is probably increased postoperatively. Heparin prophylaxis is therefore advised in the obese patient and cessation of smoking and the use of pre- and postoperative respiratory physiotherapy are also probably indicated. In extreme obesity, weight loss may be indicated both to reduce the technical problems of the surgeon and because as little as 10–15% of weight loss has been shown to have beneficial effects on cardiopulmonary and metabolic functions (Pasulka et al, 1986). It is important that weight loss does not lead to protein malnutrition however, and it needs to be closely supervised by a dietician.

PROPHYLAXIS AGAINST SEPSIS

Superficial wound infections are important to elderly surgical patients as they are uncomfortable and may prolong postoperative stay (Seymour and Pringle, 1982b). They also considerably increase the cost of surgical therapy. More serious, however, are deep-seated infections which are a major source of mortality, particularly in general surgical patients undergoing gastrointestinal surgery. An important development in prevention of postoperative sepsis in patients of all ages has been the use of prophylactic antibiotics and this will now be briefly discussed. Keighley (1988) has carried out extensive research on the use of prophylactic antibiotics and has stressed the need for clear definitions in this field. He points out that if infection is already present in a surgical patient (such as when surgery is being carried out for an abscess), then the term 'prophylactic antibiotic' should not be used. If antibiotics are given in this situation they are 'therapeutic' in nature.

The concept of using prophylactic antibiotics came from animal work where it was demonstrated that a high blood level of an antibiotic, at the time bacteria were being inoculated into a wound, was able to prevent subsequent infection. Subsequent work with humans seemed to confirm this finding, although there are still disputes about the correct antibiotics to use for different circumstances. Most regimens involve intravenous doses of antibiotics shortly before surgery (and certainly within four hours). One or two doses may also be needed after surgery or be given during particularly long surgical procedures. Many regimens have involved cephalosporins as low toxicity drugs with a wide spectrum of activity. Some recent recommendations for prophylaxis in all types of surgery have been given by Kaiser (1986). For gynaecological surgery he recommends no prophylaxis for simple dilation and curettage. For abdominal or vaginal hysterectomy, Kaiser suggests cephazolin (1 g intravenously) preoperatively and six and twelve hours later. In patients with an allergy, doxycycline (200 mg intravenously) preoperative has been used for vaginal hysterectomy.

DEEP VENOUS THROMBOSIS AND PULMONARY EMBOLISM

When special diagnostic tests are used, the incidence of postoperative deep venous thrombosis (DVT) in general surgical and gynaecological patients aged over 40 is between 10 and 45% (Rose et al, 1979; Consensus Conference, 1986). With increasing age, incidences tend to be higher and Borow and Goldson (1981) found postoperative DVTs in 65% of general surgical patients over 71. The main life-threatening consequence of a DVT is a massive pulmonary embolism (PE) which has been estimated to cause the deaths of 1% of general surgical patients if no prophylaxis is given (Kakkar et al, 1975). Kakkar and his colleagues (1969, 1975) have documented that DVTs which are confined to the calf rarely cause major PEs but that more proximal DVTs are much more hazardous.

In general surgical and low-risk gynaecology patients (see below), DVTs probably begin in the calf as the result of stasis. Low dose subcutaneous heparin appears to offer effective prophylaxis against this type of DVT (Kakkar and Adams, 1986). Such DVTs extend proximally in perhaps one fifth to a quarter of cases (Kakkar, 1969, 1975) without prophylaxis.

Added risks of PE are to be found in orthopaedic surgery and extensive pelvic survery for carcinoma. Here surgery may cause direct trauma to femoral vessels. The resulting proximal DVTs are more likely to embolize than those confined to the calf, and subcutaneous heparin may be inadequate prophylaxis (see below).

A recent Consensus Conference (1986) has been held in the USA to consider the prophylaxis of DVT and PE. Gynaecological patients were divided into three groups:

1. *Low risk* patients were defined as those under 40, having operations of 30 minutes or less. Here the risk of DVT was estimated to be less than 3% and no prophylaxis was recommended except early mobilization and antiembolism stockings.
2. *Moderate risk* patients comprised those between 40 and 70 years undergoing minor or major surgery, but with no other risk factors being present. Here the risk of DVT is 10–40% and the recommendations for prophylaxis were low dose subcutaneous heparin and/or external pneumatic compression of the calf. Dextran was also suggested as an alternative.
3. *High risk* patients were defined as those over 40 who had added risk factors such as previous DVT/PE, varicose veins, infection, malignancy, oestrogen therapy, obesity and prolonged surgery. Here the risk of DVT is 40–70% and there is a 1–5% risk of fatal PE. For non-malignant high-risk cases the Consensus Conference recommendations for prophylaxis were the same as for moderate risk patients. Where malignancy was present, however, then dextran and/or external pneumatic compression was recommended. Low-dose heparin plus external pneumatic compression was mentioned as a possible alternative as was full anticoagulation with warfarin.

In the future, multiple regression equations may allow us to predict postoperative thromboembolism with greater precision, perhaps allowing for more selective use of prophylaxis. Two important papers in this respect are those by Crandon et al (1980a,b). A recent report has attempted to predict postoperative DVT using clinical preoperative findings only (Clarke-Pearson et al, 1987). If this prognostic model maintains its predictive value in a new set of patients, it may prove useful in day to day clinical practice.

PROBLEMS OF FLUID BALANCE, AND RENAL INSUFFICIENCY

Glomerular filtration rate tends to fall by 4–8 ml/min for each decade after the age of 40, although there is a wide degree of variability (Lindemann, 1975; Samiy, 1983). This implies that many, although not all, elderly patients will need reduced doses of those drugs (such as digoxin or gentamicin) which are primarily excreted by the kidneys (Seymour, 1986). The *British National Formulary* gives recommendations of drug doses both in the elderly and in the presence of renal impairment, and should be consulted in individual cases.

Salt and volume depletion may be difficult to detect in the elderly patient (Table 3). While the gynaecological surgeon is less likely to encounter massive volume depletion than is the general surgeon admitting 'acute

Table 3. Clinical signs of salt and water depletion in the old and young. From Seymour and Vaz (1987), with permission.

'Textbook' signs	Problems of interpretation in the elderly
Cardiovascular	
Postural hypotension	Common even in fit elderly
Supine hypotension	May be masked by pre-existing systolic hypertension
Tachycardia	Maximal heart rate less in elderly
Cold extremities, cutaneous lividity	Valid in young and old, but late sign
Reduced pulmonary wedge pressure (Swan–Ganz)	Valid, but invasive
Absence of peripheral oedema	Valid, but note local causes of ankle oedema in elderly
Tissue changes	
Dry tongue	Unreliable sign at any age
Reduced tongue volume	Difficult to quantify
Reduced skin turgor	Skin elasticity falls with age
Sunken eyes	Valid, but very late sign
Miscellaneous	
Oliguria	May be less marked in elderly as a degree of renal insufficiency is common
Drowsiness, apathy	Non-specific signs

abdomens', particular attention needs to be paid to elderly patients on chronic diuretic therapy or those who have voluntarily restricted their fluid intake because of incontinence.

Volume depletion is an accepted risk factor for postoperative acute renal failure and intraoperative hypotension. Nephrotoxic drugs may add to the risk and a full list (which includes many antibiotics, diuretics and non-steroidal anti-inflammatory agents) is given by Seymour (1986). While patients with chronic renal failure need careful assessment prior to surgery, they are not usually volume-depleted, and postoperative problems tend to be few as long as the renal status is taken into account when prescribing drugs.

The elderly kidney, even in an apparently fit person, may be less efficient in concentrating urine and diluting urine than the kidney of a younger patient. The risk of volume depletion and overload is thus increased and prescription of postoperative intravenous fluids needs to be based on a constant assessment of the individual patient, rather than on 'standard' postoperative fluid regimens (Seymour, 1986).

THE USE OF ROUTINE PREOPERATIVE TESTS

The use of 'routine' preoperative haematological, biochemical, and radio-logical tests in young general surgical patients is being increasingly criticized by investigators who have found that such tests rarely influence surgical management (Fowkes, 1985; Kaplan et al, 1985; Muskett and McGreevy, 1986; McKee and Scott, 1987). However, few of these studies have considered older patients, where the incidence of disease tends to be higher and where atypical presentation of disease is common. McKee and Scott (1987), while showing a low yield of routine tests in younger surgical patients, nevertheless suggested a full blood count for patients over 40, a urea and electrolytes for patients over 60 having major surgery, an ECG for all patients over 50 and a chest X-ray for those over 60 having major surgery. Our own experience supports the above policy (Seymour et al, 1982, 1983) and we would also recommend a blood sugar in all preoperative elderly patients. Where there is a strong chance of malignancy or where there are unexplained vague symptoms we find that calcium and liver function tests may help in the preoperative assessment. A thyroid function test should also be considered in patients with lethargy, recent weight alteration, or intolerance of cold or heat.

When specific studies become available in elderly gynaecological patients, these recommendations may need to be modified.

REFERENCES

Andersen B & Ostberg J (1972) Survival rates in surgery of the aged. Assessment of long-term prognosis according to co-existing disease. *Gerontologia Clinica* **14:** 354–360.

Babu SC, Sharma PVP, Raciti A et al (1980) Monitor-guided responses. Operability with safety is increased in patients with peripheral vascular diseases. *Archives of Surgery* **115:** 1384–1386.

Bartlett RH (1980) Pulmonary pathophysiology in surgical patients. *Surgery Clinics of North America* **60:** 1323–1338.

Bastow MD, Rawlings J & Allison SP (1983) Benefits of supplementary tube feeding after fractured neck of femur: a randomised controlled trial. *British Medical Journal* **287:** 1589–1592.

Becker R (1986) Cardiac Risk in Non-Cardiac Surgery. *Annals of Internal Medicine* **104:** 887.

Becker RC & Underwood DA (1987) Myocardial infarction in patients undergoing non-cardiac surgery. *Cleveland Clinic Journal of Medicine* **54:** 25–28.

Bedford PD (1955) Adverse cerebral effects of anaesthesia on old people. *Lancet* **ii:** 259–263.

Borow M & Goldson H (1981) Post-operative venous thrombosis. Evaluation of five methods of treatment. *American Journal of Surgery* **141:** 245–251.

Boucher CA, Brewster DC, Darling RC, Okada RD, Strauss HW & Pohost GM (1985) Determination of cardiac risk by dipyridamole-thallium imaging before peripheral vascular surgery. *New England Journal of Medicine* **312:** 389–394.

Boyd JB, Bradford B & Watne AL (1980) Operative risk factors of colon resection in the elderly. *Annals of Surgery* **192:** 743–746.

Buck N, Devlin HB & Lunn JN (1987) Report of a Confidential Enquiry into Perioperative Deaths (CEPOD), London: Nuffield Provincial Hospital Trust.

Burns HJG (1988) Nutritional support in the perioperative period. *British Medical Bulletin* **44:** 357–373.

Caird FI & Akhtar AJ (1972) Chronic respiratory disease in the elderly. A population study. *Thorax* **27:** 764–768.

Castillo R & Haas A (1985) Chest physical therapy: comparative efficacy of pre-operative and post-operative in the elderly. *Archives of Physical Medicine and Rehabilitation* **66:** 376–379.

Clarke-Pearson DL, DeLong ER, Synan IS, Coleman RE & Creasman WJ (1987) Variables associated with post-operative deep venous thrombosis: a prospective study of 411 gynaecology patients and creation of a prognostic model. *Obstetrics and Gynecology* **69:** 146–150.

Clinch D, Banerjee AK & Ostick G (1984) Absence of pain in elderly patients with peptic ulcer. *Age and Ageing* **13:** 120–123.

Consensus Conference (1986) Prevention of venous thrombosis and pulmonary embolism.

Journal of the American Medical Association **256:** 744–749.

Coriat P, Fauchet M, Bousseau D et al (1985) Left ventricular dysfunction after non-cardiac surgical procedures in patients with ischemic heart disease. *Acta Anaesthesiologica Scandinavica* **29:** 804–810.

Corman LC (1979) The pre-operative patient with an asymptomatic cervical bruit. *Medical Clinics of North America* **63:** 1335–1340.

Cotes JE (1979) *Lung Function Assessment and Application in Medicine*, 4th edn. London: Blackwell Scientific Publications.

Crandon AJ, Peel KR, Anderson JA, Thompson V & McNicol GP (1980a) Post-operative deep vein thrombosis: identifying high-risk patients. *British Medical Journal* **281:** 343–344.

Crandon AJ, Peel KR, Anderson JA, Thompson V & McNicol GP (1980b) Prophylaxis of post-operative deep vein thrombosis: elective use of low-dose heparin in high-risk patients. *British Medical Journal* **281:** 345–347.

Del Guercio LRM & Cohn JD (1980) Monitoring operative risks in the elderly. *Journal of the American Medical Association* **243:** 1350–1355.

Detsky AS, Abrams HB, McLaughlin JR et al (1986a) Predicting cardiac complications in patients undergoing non-cardiac surgery. *Journal of General Internal Medicine* **1:** 211–219.

Detsky AS, Abrams HB, Forbath N, Scott JG & Hilliard JR (1986b) Cardiac assessment for patients undergoing non-cardiac surgery. A multifactorial clinical risk index. *Archives of Internal Medicine* **146:** 2131–2134.

Detsky AS, Baker JP, O'Rourke KO et al (1987) Predicting nutrition-associated complications for patients undergoing gastro-intestinal surgery. *Journal of Parenteral and Enteral Nutrition* **11:** 440–446.

Farrow SC, Fowkes FGR, Lunn JN, Robertson IB & Samuel P (1982) Epidemiology in Anaesthesia II. Factors affecting mortality in hospital. *British Journal of Anaesthesia* **54:** 811–816.

Fenyo G (1974) Diagnostic problems of acute abdominal diseases in the aged. *Acta Chirurgica Scandinavica* **140:** 396–405.

Fowkes FGR (1985) Containing the use of diagnostic tests. *British Medical Journal* **290:** 488–489.

Fowkes FG, Lunn JN, Farrow SC, Robertson IB & Samuel P (1982) Epidemiology in Anaesthesia III. Mortality risk in patients with co-existing physical disease. *British Journal of Anaesthesia* **54:** 819–825.

Gardner TJ, Horneffer PJ, Manolio TA et al (1985) Stroke following coronary artery bypass grafting: a ten-year study. *Annals of Thoracic Surgery* **40:** 574–580.

Garibaldi RA, Britt MR, Coleman ML, Reading JC & Pace NL (1981) Risk factors for post-operative pneumonia. *American Journal of Medicine* **70:** 677–680.

Gass GD & Olsen GN (1986) Pre-operative pulmonary function testing to predict post-operative morbidity and mortality. *Chest* **89:** 127–135.

Gerson MC, Hurst JM, Hertzberg VS et al (1985) Cardiac prognosis in non-cardiac geriatric surgery. *Annals of Internal Medicine* **103** (6, part 1): 832–837.

Goldman L & Caldera DL (1979) Risk of general anaesthesia and elective operation in the hypertensive patient. *Anaesthesia* **50:** 285–292.

Goldman L, Caldera DL, Nussbaum SR et al (1977) Multifactorial index of cardiac risk in non-cardiac surgical procedures. *New England Journal of Medicine* **297:** 845–850.

Gray GE & Gray LK (1979) Validity of anthropometric norms used in the assessment of hospitalised patients. *Journal of Parenteral and Enteral Nutrition* **3:** 366–368.

Greenburg AG, Salk RP, Coyle JJ & Peskin GW (1981) Mortality and gastro-intestinal surgery in the elderly. Elective versus emergency procedures. *Archives of Surgery* **116:** 788–791.

Hedley-Whyte J, Burgess GE, Feeley TW & Miller MG (1976) *Applied Physiology of Respiratory Care*. Boston: Little Brown and Company.

Hill GL (1987) Malnutrition and surgical risk: guidelines for nutritional therapy. *Annals of the Royal College of Surgeons of England* **69:** 263–265.

Jaluvka V (1980) Surgical geriatric gynaecology. A contribution to geriatric gynecology with particular consideration of post-operative mortality *Gynecology and Obstetrics*, vol. 7.

Jeejeebhoy KN & Meguid MM (1986) Assessment of nutritional status in the oncologic patient. *Surgical Clinics of North America* **66:** 1077–1090.

Jeffrey CC, Kunsman J, Cullen DJ & Brewster DC (1983) A prospective evaluation of cardiac risk index. *Anesthesiology* **58:** 462–464.

Kaiser AB (1986) Antimicrobial prophylaxis in surgery. *New England Journal of Medicine* **315**: 1129–1138.

Kakkar VV & Adams PC (1986) Preventive and therapeutic approach to venous thrombo-embolic disease and pulmonary embolism—can death from pulmonary embolism be prevented? *Journal of the American College of Cardiology* **8**: 146B–158B.

Kakkar VV, Howe CT, Flanc C & Clarke MB (1969) Natural history of post-operative deep vein thrombosis. *Lancet* **ii**: 230–233.

Kakkar VV, Corrigan TB & Fossard DP (1975) Prevention of fatal post-operative pulmonary embolism by low doses of heparin. An international multi-centre trial. *Lancet* **ii**: 45–51.

Kaplan EB, Sheiner LB, Boeckmann AJ et al (1985) The usefulness of pre-operative laboratory screening. *Journal of the American Medical Association* **253**: 3576–3581.

Keighley MRB (1988) Infection: prophylaxis. *British Medical Bulletin* **44**: 374–402.

Knapp WS, Douglas JS, Craver JM et al (1981) Efficacy of coronary artery bypass grafting in elderly patients with coronary artery disease. *American Journal of Cardiology* **47**: 923–930.

Larsen SF, Olesen KH, Jacobsen E et al (1987) Prediction of cardiac risk in non-cardiac surgery. *European Heart Journal* **8**: 179–185.

Lewis FR (1980) Management of atelectasis and pneumonia. *Surgical Clinics of North America* **60**: 1391–1401.

Lindemann PD (1975) Age changes in renal function. In Goldmann R & Rockstein M (eds). *The Physiology and Pathology of Human Ageing*. New York: Academic Press.

Lipowski ZJ (1980) *Delirium. Acute Brain Failure in Man*. Springfield, Illinois: CC Thomas.

Loeb HS, Reid R, Pifarre R, Gunnar RM & Scanlon PJ (1985) Usefulness of post-operative enzymes for diagnosis of perioperative myocardial infarction following aortocoronary bypass. *Acute Care* **11**: 40–47.

McKee RF & Scott EM (1987) The value of routine pre-operative investigations. *Annals of the Royal College of Surgeons of England* **69**: 160–162.

Masey SA & Burton GW (1987) Anaesthesia for patients with cardiac disease. Pre-operative management. *British Journal of Hospital Medicine* **37**: 386–396.

Merli GJ & Weitz HH (eds) (1987) Pre-operative consultation. *Medical Clinics of North America* **71**: 353–585.

Mlynek HJ, Hartig W, Schenker V & Winiecki P (1977) Komplikationen und Gefahren bein abdominalen chirugischen Erkrankungen im Senium. *Zentralblatt Für Chirurgie* **102**: 283–296.

Morise AP, McDowell DE, Savrin RA et al (1987) The prediction of cardiac risk in patients undergoing vascular surgery. *American Journal of Medical Science* **293**: 150–158.

Muskett AD & McGreevy JM (1986) Rational pre-operative evaluation. *Postgraduate Medical Journal* **62**: 925–928.

Norman J, Lorimer AR, Grenfell A & Mansell MA (1988) Pre-operative patient assessment. *British Medical Bulletin* **42**: 247–268.

Noviant Y, Silbert D, Capdevielle G, Langloys J (1976) Etude de quelques éléments d'évaluation du risque respiratoire post-operatoire chez le sujet agé. *Anesthésie Analgésie Réanimation* **33**: 285–295.

O'Donohue WJ (1985a) Prevention and treatment of post-operative atelectasis. Can it and will it be adequately studied? *Chest* **87**: 1–3.

O'Donohue WJ (1985b) National survey of the usage of lung expansion modalities for the prevention and treatment of post-operative atelectasis following abdominal and thoracic surgery. *Chest* **87**: 76–80.

Palmberg S & Hirsjarvi E (1979) Mortality in geriatric surgery. *Gerontology* **25**: 103–112.

Pasulka PS, Bistrian BR, Benotti PN & Blackburn GL (1986) The risks of surgery in obese patients. *Annals of Internal Medicine* **104**: 540–546.

Peters RM (1979) Pulmonary physiologic studies of the perioperative period. *Chest* **76**: 576–584.

Prys-Roberts C (1979) Hypertension and anesthesia—fifty years on. *Anesthesiology* **50**: 281–284.

Rees JL (1982) Accuracy of hospital activity analysis data in estimating the incidence of proximal femoral fracture. *British Medical Journal* **284**: 1856–1857.

Reiss R, Deutsch AA, Nudelman I. (1987) Abdominal surgery in elderly patients: statistical analysis of clinical factors prognostic of mortality of 1000 cases. *Mount Sinai Journal of Medicine* **54**: 135–140.

Rose SD, Corman LC & Mason DT (1979) Cardiac risk factors in patients undergoing non-cardiac surgery. *Medical Clinics of North America* **63**: 1271–1288.

Samiy AH (1983) Renal disease in the elderly. *Medical Clinics of North America* **67**: 463–480.

Seymour DG (1986) Medical Assessment of the Elderly Surgical Patient, pp 3, 127, 137–170, 150–155, 168, 190, 200, 210–219. London: Croom Helm.

Seymour DG (1988) *Prediction of Risk in the Elderly Surgical Patient*. MD Thesis, University of Birmingham.

Seymour DG & Pringle R (1982a) A new method of auditing surgical mortality rates: application to a group of elderly general surgical patients. *British Medical Journal* **284**: 1539–1542.

Seymour DG & Pringle R (1982b) Elderly patients in a general surgical unit: do they block beds? *British Medical Journal* **284**: 1921–1923.

Seymour DG & Pringle R (1983) Post-operative complications in the elderly surgical patient. *Gerontology* **29**: 262–270.

Seymour DG & Seymour RM (1988) The physiology of ageing. In Pathy MSJ & Finucane P (eds) *Practical Geriatric Medicine*. London: Springer-Verlag.

Seymour DG & Vaz FG (1987) Aspects of surgery in the aged: pre-operative medical assessment. *British Journal of Hospital Medicine* **37**: 102–112.

Seymour DG, Pringle R & Shaw JW (1982) The role of the routine pre-operative chest X-ray in the elderly general surgical patient. *Postgraduate Medical Journal* **58**: 741–745.

Seymour DG, Pringle R & MacLennan WJ (1983) The role of the routine pre-operative electrocardiogram in the elderly surgical patient. *Age and Ageing* **12**: 97–104.

Shaw PJ, Bates D, Cartlidge NE et al (1987) Neurologic and neuropsychological morbidity following major surgery: comparison of coronary artery bypass and peripheral vascular surgery. *Stroke* **18**: 700–707.

Sherlock DJ, Randle J, Playforth M, Cox R & Holl-Allen RTJ (1984) Can nocturnal emergency surgery be reduced? *British Medical Journal* **289**: 170–171.

Simpson BR, Williams M, Scott JF & Crampton Smith A (1961) The effects of anaesthesia and elective surgery in old people. *Lancet* **ii**: 887–893.

Slogoff S & Keats AS (1985) Does perioperative myocardial ischemia lead to post-operative myocardial infarction? *Anesthesiology* **62**: 107–114.

Smith PLC, Treasure T, Newman SP et al (1986) Cerebral consequences of cardiopulmonary bypass. *Lancet* **i**: 823–825.

Starker PM, La Sala PA, Askanazi J, Todd G, Hensle TW & Kinney JM (1986) The influence of pre-operative total parenteral nutrition upon morbidity and mortality. *Surgery, Gynecology and Obstetrics* **162**: 569–574.

Stephen CR (1986) Risk factors and outcome in elderly patients: an epidemiologic study. In Stephen CR & Assaf RAE (eds) *Geriatric Anesthesia: Principles and Practice*, pp 345–362. Boston: Butterworths.

Stock MC, Downs JB, Gauer PK, Alster JM & Imrey PB (1985) Prevention of post-operative pulmonary complications with CPAP, incentive spirometry and conservative therapy. *Chest* **87**: 151–157.

Tisi GM (1979) Pre-operative evaluation of pulmonary function. *American Review of Respiratory Disease* **119**: 293–310.

Tisi GM (1987) Pre-operative identification and evaluation of the patient with lung disease. *Medical Clinics of North America* **71**: 399–412.

Vaz FG & Seymour DG (1988) A prospective study of elderly general surgical patients in Cardiff. Methodology and pre-operative problems (submitted for publication).

Waters J, Wilkinson C, Golmon M, Schoeppels S, Linde HW & Brunner EA (1981) Evaluation of cardiac risk in non-cardiac surgical patients. *Anesthesiology* **55**: A343.

Whates PD, Birzgalis AR & Irving M (1982) Accuracy of hospital activity analysis operation codes. *British Medical Journal* **284**: 1857–1858.

Wilcutts HD (1977) Nutritional assessment of 1000 surgical patients in an affluent suburban community hospital. *Journal of Parenteral and Enteral Nutrition* **1**: 25A.

Yousif H, Davies G, Westaby S, Prendiville OF, Sapsford RN & Oakley CM (1987) Pre-operative myocardial ischaemia: its relation to perioperative infarction. *British Heart Journal* **58**: 9–14.

4

Menopause—a multi system disease

MARK BRINCAT
JOHN W. W. STUDD

An astonishing omission from current textbooks of geriatric medicine is reference to the endocrinopathy of the menopause and the treatment or prevention of many of the infirmities of old age with oestrogens. The population is ageing as the total lifespan of women has gradually increased. At the time of the Roman Empire, the average life expectancy of women was only 23 years (Schneider, 1986). From the Middle Ages until the late nineteenth century, fewer than 30% of women reached the menopause. Today with the average life expectancy of women being 78 years, there are just under ten million post-menopausal women in the United Kingdom and 40 million in the United States. This contributes to 17% of the total population.

Women now spend 30% of their lives after the menopause in a state of profound oestrogen deprivation. The realization of the profound changes that occur as a result of this ovarian failure and the relatively simple treatments that are available for the condition make it imperative that more effort should be dedicated to the study of the post-menopausal years with specialist clinics being more widely available to women.

AGE OF ONSET

The average age of the menopause has not changed over the centuries. Amudsen and Diers (1973) quote several authors who all give the average age of the menopause at around 50. Amongst these are; Aristotle (50) (sixth century AD), Paulus Aegineta (50) (seventh century AD), Hildegrad (50) (twelfth century AD), Gilbertus Anglicus (50) (thirteenth century AD). At present the average age of the menopause has been estimated as being 51 years.

Thus the age of the menopause does not appear to be related to the age of menarche, socio-economic factors, race, poverty, weight or height. The only factor that apparently may influence the age of onset of the menopause is cigarette smoking which lowers it (Frie, 1980; Wilson et al, 1985). Race does not seem to influence the real age of the menopause. McKinlay et al

(1972) report the same menopausal age in caucasians as Frere (1971) does in South African black women.

DEFINITIONS

The *climacteric* is commonly referred to as that period of time around the menopause when ovarian function is erratic, with partial gonadal failure occurring in the two to three year transitional phase during which reproduction ceases. This is a time of decreasing fertility, decreasing plasma oestrogen levels and the appearance of the typical symptoms of the menopausal syndrome, although of course the menstrual periods will still be present.

The *menopause* is the one fixed event of the climacteric. This refers to the last menstrual bleed and subsequent unscheduled vaginal bleeding must be regarded as an abnormality which requires investigation. The menopause is generally considered to have occurred retrospectively after one year of amenorrhoea.

PATHOPHYSIOLOGY

The ageing of the ovary with a progressive decrease in the number of follicles begins even before birth (Baker, 1963). The percentage of growing follicles markedly increases at puberty and is maintained through most of the reproductive life but decreases markedly at the menopause.

The mean weight of the ovary begins to decrease at the age of 30 (Nocke, 1986). Table 1 gives a summary of the endocrine changes that occur at the climacteric. A detailed description is beyond the scope of this chapter.

Table 1. Summary of endocrine changes at the climacteric.

Phase I. Hypothalamic–pituitary hyperactivity
Starts 10–15 years before menopause
Compensatory for increased resistance of ovarian follicles and decreased follicular hormone secretion
Evidenced by raised FSH and, later LH–pituitary may become exhausted late post-menopause

Phase II. Ovulation and corpus luteum failure
Occurs in most women with increasing frequency as menopause approaches—anovulatory cycles or shortened luteal phase
Deficient progesterone and continued unopposed oestrogen secretion
Causes dysfunctional uterine bleeding, endometrial hyperplasia and carcinoma

Phase III. Ovarian follicular failure
Failure of follicular development causes fall in oestradiol secretion and cessation of menses
Ovarian stroma remains active; with adrenal cortex, produces androstenedione and testosterone
Oestrone produced by extraglandular conversion of androgens is the main post-menopausal oestrogen—only 10–50% of post-menopausal women are oestrogen deficient.

CONSEQUENCES OF OVARIAN FAILURE

The primary causative deficiency that leads to the clinical consequences of ovarian failure is that of oestrogen deficiency. The high levels of follicle stimulating hormone (FSH) and luteinizing hormone (LH) are irrelevant to the production of symptoms but a single plasma FSH level of >15 iu/litre would be diagnostic of the menopausal state (Chakravati et al, 1976).

The well recognized reduction in bone mass, the development of what are currently regarded as adverse changes in blood lipid lipoprotein concentration, the generalized atrophy of all connective tissues, (although only obvious several years after the onset of the menopause) can be directly attributable to oestrogen deficiency.

There are other more immediate symptoms associated with the climacteric referred to collectively as the 'menopausal syndrome'. This term describes various physical and psychological symptoms which certain women develop and once again it would seem that it is ovarian failure that contributes to this condition. Because this syndrome can predate the menopause, however, the various symptoms of the syndrome can also be attributable to fluctuating levels of sex steroids and gonadotrophins although the exact relationship between the two remains unclear. Table 2 indicates the climacteric symptoms of the syndrome.

Table 2. Frequency of complaints in menopausal women, ages 45–54 years.

Complaint	Number of women (%)
Irritability	92
Lethargy/fatigue	88
Depression	78
Headaches	71
Hot flushes	68
Forgetfulness	64
Weight gain	61
Insomnia	51
Joint pain/backache	48
Palpitations	44
Crying spells	42
Constipation	37
Dysuria	20
Decreased libido	20

SHORT-TERM CONSEQUENCES

The short-term symptoms of the menopause that have been documented are numerous. Table 2 indicates the commonest ones presenting in the immediate post-menopausal period. Many of these short-term (immediate) symptoms were shown to be present in a group of young women following hysterectomy and bilateral oophorectomy (Chakravarti et al, 1976) and another group who had been subjected to radiation menopause of their ovaries as a result of radiotherapy for acute myeloid leukaemia (Whitehead and Crust, 1987).

The short-term consequences of the menopause are divided for convenience into sympathetic or vasomotor symptoms, end organ atrophy and psychological symptoms.

Vasomotor instability

The hot flush is the most characteristic, but not necessarily the most common, symptom of the menopause with 50–70% of women in the climacteric and in their post-menopausal years complaining of the symptom, (McKinlay and Jeffreys, 1974) and 20–25% of women still complaining of these symptoms five years later (Thompson et al, 1973).

Hot flushes may occur at any time of the day or night and can be triggered by a variety of common situations such as sleeping or dozing, work activities, recreation and relaxation or housework. In a survey of 20 subjects with frequent flushes, Voda (1981) found that of 974 events that were recorded as preceding a hot flush, sleep related activities were the highest and 'emotions' the lowest. Prodromal symptoms are common and for many can include a feeling of increasing pressure in the head, though most women have difficulty in describing the sensation (Tataryn et al, 1980). During the night, a decrease of rapid eye movement (REM) sleep and waking often precedes a hot flush (Erlik et al, 1981).

With most women, a flush starts in the face, neck, head or chest and the initial focal point may be very specific: ear lobe, forehead, or between the breasts. Subsequent spread of the sensation to the head may be in any direction. The duration of a flush can last from a few seconds up to an hour and there is a large variation in the frequency of flushes (Sturdee et al, 1978; Voda, 1981). The more intense and severe flushing episodes may be followed by sweating, although some also will sweat without an apparent initial flush. When these episodes occur during the night they might lead to insomnia. These episodes may also be coupled with irritability and general lethargy. All these associated symptoms have been shown repeatedly to respond to successful treatment of flushes (Campbell and Whitehead, 1977; Brincat et al, 1984a,b).

Aetiology

Although flushes are the most characteristic symptom of the menopause, very little is known about their aetiology. The precise role that oestrogens play has yet to be established but explanations relying on a mechanism by raised gonadotrophins alone causing flushes are almost certainly wrong because flushes occur with great severity in women who have had a hypophysectomy or who are on luteinizing hormone releasing hormone (LHRH) agonists (Lightman et al, 1982).

All the major sex steroids, androgens, oestrogens and progestogens seem to play a part. Flushes have been reported in orchidectomized men and testosterone replacement by IM injections every 2–4 weeks eliminates flushes in such men and restores libido and potency (Fieldman et al, 1976; Hendy and Burge, 1983; De Fazio et al, 1984). These flushes are indistinguishable from those in hypo-oestrogenaemic women. Flushes respond well to treatment with gestogens (Appleby, 1962; Schiff et al, 1980; Patterson, 1982).

Flushes do not seem to be isolated events. Peripheral vascular control is poor after the menopause and reactions to stimuli are damaged (Figure 1). This peripheral vascular control can be restored by the use of oestrogens (Brincat et al, 1984a). Poor peripheral vascular control occurs in hypo-oestrogenaemic women regardless of whether flushes are present or not and, thus, flushes appear to be the result of a total breakdown in peripheral vascular control leading to a massive vasodilatation, followed by a vaso-constriction, in response to some stimulus (Brincat et al, 1984a).

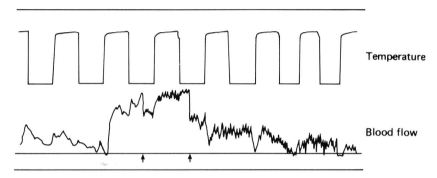

Figure 1. A hot flush occurring in an untreated patient during thermal entainment testing whilst applying a hot and cold stimulus alternating every 40 s (top trace). The first part of the bottom trace shows poor peripheral vascular control as measured by photoplathysmography. The hot flush begins coincident with a hot stimulus (elevation and thicker trace—bottom). The base line had to be changed twice (arrows) so as to keep the trace within the confines of the recording paper. From Brincat et al (1984).

These vasomotor symptoms have a particular importance in older women. The night sweats produce insomnia with lethargy and loss of con-centration during the day. They are often manifested by giddiness and falling attacks, which may have the disastrous consequence of femoral neck fractures in women with osteoporosis. Thus oestrogens are of great import-ance not only in the prevention of osteoporosis but in the prevention of the minor falls which lead to major pathology.

End organ atrophy

Patients can present with vaginal dryness leading to dyspareunia, apareunia and recurrent vaginal infections.

The genital tract and the urethra have a common embryological origin and oestrogen deficiency thus will affect both systems. Recurrent urinary infections may occur and atrophy of the urethra and the trigone of the bladder may be the cause in the elderly woman of the common symptoms of dysuria, frequency, urgency (i.e. the urethral syndrome; Smith, 1972).

Psychological changes

Anxiety, irritability and depression arising in association with vasomotor and atrophic symptoms are common around the time of the menopause (Campbell, 1975; Studd and Parsons, 1977; Studd et al, 1977; Dennerstein and Burrows; 1978; Brincat et al, 1984b) and are often at their most severe in the year or two before the periods cease.

Although vasomotor and atrophic symptoms are generally attributed to hormonal changes and can be treated with oestrogen therapy, no such agreement exists about the frequency and aetiology of psychiatric disturbances. Double blind trials have shown the beneficial effects of oestrogen therapy on psychiatric disturbances (Campbell, 1975; Thombom and Oswald, 1977), but these studies have been criticized for their poor definition of the post-menopausal status and the use of non-standardized psychological tests (Dennerstein and Burrows, 1978).

Montgomery et al (1987) published an important work on the subject using a standardized method of psychiatric assessment. The women analysed were attending the Dulwich Menopause Clinic and results must therefore be interpreted as applying to a select group. Nevertheless, it was an unexpected finding that of these women, in many cases not attending the clinic for primary psychological symptoms, 86% had clinical psychiatric illness. This was a much greater proportion than other reports of 29% of women aged 40–55 with clinical psychiatric illness in a general population sample (Ballinger, 1975) and 52% of women of a similar age, referred to a gynaecological clinic largely due to menstrual abnormalities (Ballinger, 1977).

As yet no clinical link between the menopause and depression has been established. The highest incidence of depression in middle life arises in the few years before the cessation of periods (Jazsman, 1973). The suggestion is, therefore, that it is not low level of oestrogens, but changes in hormone concentration, such as those in the cyclical depression of pre-menstrual syndrome (Magos et al, 1986), that predispose to depression during the menopause. There is evidence that women who are depressed are those who are most anxious about the menopause and attribute their low mood to it.

A possible mechanism for the increase in psychological problems around the time of the menopause could be the interaction that exists between oestrogens and various control neurotransmitters. Falling oestrogen levels may lead to low activity of control nervous system transmitters, either by reducing available tryptophan for serotonin synthesis or by reducing dopamine receptor sensitivity (Aylward, 1975).

The physical symptoms of the menopause may cause a secondary depression in some susceptible women. Alternatively, the loss of reproductive potential may be seen as a loss of femininity and result in low esteem. This loss of femininity, as described by women, is not unique to late post-menopausal women but has also been described in women with early menopause such as those studied by Whitehead and Crust (1987).

Depression is at least twice as common in women than men and as this difference only begins with puberty and is associated with the pre-menstrual state and the post-natal state as well as the post-menopausal years, it is believed by many to be the result of either deficiency or sudden changes in plasma oestradiol levels. An alternative point of view is that the excess of depression in women is an environmental factor related to the middle-aged woman's role in society and not in any way related to gonadal hormones. The sad sequel to this is that approximately 40% of women in this age group are taking tranquillizers and antidepressants instead of replacement oestrogens. This results in more depression, addiction to cycloactive drugs and yet more dizziness and falling attacks which might be the fatal endpoint of post-menopausal osteoporosis.

Libido and lethargy

Loss of libido and lethargy are two other common psychological symptoms attributed to the menopause (Neugarten and Kraines, 1965). Distinction needs to be made between dyspareunia and loss of libido. Accurate diagnosis is essential because symptoms resulting from domestic problems are best treated by psychiatrists, marriage guidance counsellors or social workers. The loss of libido that is associated with the menopause is characteristically a loss of interest in normal sexual relations in the presence of an otherwise happy marriage (Studd and Parsons, 1977; Studd et al, 1977; Sarrel, 1988).

Psychosexual symptoms have proved very difficult to study because of the lack of objective analysis for carrying out libido studies. Montgomery et al (personal communication) have looked at the problem using an objective assessment and has established that loss of libido is indeed a feature of the post-menopausal years. As with lethargy (Brincat, 1984b) they have found that good responses can be achieved with adequate hormone replacement, although the role of additional testosterone is still debatable.

LONG-TERM CONSEQUENCES

The long-term consequences of ovarian failure carry a high morbidity and mortality. There is increasing evidence that with appropriate hormone replacement these can be prevented to varying degrees. New insights are being obtained into the protective influence of the female sex hormones against cardiovascular disease. The other long-term consequences that will be dealt with here are different facets of a general decrease and derangement in connective tissue after the menopause. The most important manifestations of this connective tissue disorder are in bones (osteoporosis), skin and bladder.

Short-term consequences should perhaps be more appropriately referred to as immediate consequences, as there is no evidence that peripheral vascular control gets any better with increasing age, even though flushes might subside. Likewise end organ atrophy and to some extent psychological disturbances that are due to ovarian failure are not limiting. Women learn to live with their handicap!

Cardiovascular disease

Prior to the menopause, ischaemic heart disease is uncommon in women who do not smoke, have hypertension or diabetes mellitus. Heart disease is five times more common in men than pre-menopausal women. Following the menopause, however, there is an increase in the incidence of this condition so that by the age of 70 there is no longer any sex difference. The timing of this increase in heart disease in women strongly suggests that the oestrogen deficiency of the menopause is responsible. The precise mechanism by which this is brought about remains unclear. Although it is widely believed that the menopause results in the adverse effect on the cardiovascular system through the lipoprotein metabolism, there is convincing evidence that increased low density lipoprotein (LDL) concentrations will result in increased heart disease and that increased high density lipoprotein (HDL) concentrations are cardioprotective (Gordon et al, 1977). The risk factor is expressed as the HDL/LDL ratio. Prior to the menopause the serum levels of LDL cholesterol are lower in women than in men and serum HDL is higher in pre-menopausal women as compared to men. After the menopause there is an increase in the serum HDL level in women although this does not exceed the levels in age-matched men. It appears, therefore, that in pre-menopausal women ovarian oestrogens have a protective effect against cardiovascular disease mediated by the effect on lipoprotein metabolism. It is possible that other mechanisms may also affect the role of the menopause on heart disease. Oestrogens may have a direct effect on the blood vessels and may stimulate the release of peptides which are important vasodilators. Stress may be a risk factor in heart disease, so the various symptoms of menopause such as irritability, depression and sleeplessness may be important in the increased incidence of heart disease.

The effects of hormone replacement therapy on cardiovascular disease

A number of studies have demonstrated a reduction in incidence of ischaemic heart disease following the use of hormone replacement therapy (Hammond et al, 1979; Ross et al, 1981; Stampfer et al, 1985; Bush et al, 1987). However, one smaller study by Wilson et al (1985) has disagreed with this.

Oestrogen replacement therapy causes an increase in HDL and a lowering of LDL concentrations (Figure 2; Tikkannen et al, 1986; Crook et al, 1988). These effects appear to occur after the first pass of the hormone through the liver and may not be as marked if therapy is administered parenterally. The synthetic oestrogens such as those used in the oral contraceptive pill are known to have a marked effect on the clotting system and lead to an increased risk of thromboembolic phenomena. However, the natural oestrogens used for hormone replacement therapy do not suffer from this

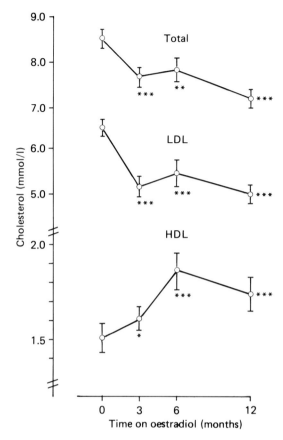

Figure 2. Effect of oestradiol valerate 2 mg/day on serum lipoprotein lipids in postmenopausal women (mean ± SD, $n = 30$). * $p < 0.02$, ** $p < 0.005$, *** $p < 0.001$. From Tikkanen et al (1985).

disadvantage. Neither do natural oestrogens affect blood pressure or carbohydrate metabolism (Thom et al, 1977, 1978). Cyclical administration of progestogens of between 7 and 13 days, in conjunction with continuous oestrogen, are essential for the prevention of endometrial hyperplasia (Studd et al, 1980). However, the progestogens may have an adverse effect on lipoprotein and carbohydrate metabolism as well as on mood (Magos et al, 1985). See below for a further discussion of this.

Osteoporosis

Peak bone mass is reached in the fourth decade of life, after which there is an age-related bone loss in both sexes. However, in women there is an acceleration in the rate of bone loss following the menopause: by the age of 70 years a woman loses 50% of her bone mass while a man loses only 25% by the age of 90 (Gordan, 1984). As a result of post-menopausal osteoporosis the fracture rate in post-menopausal women is greater than in age-matched men. It was first recognized by Bruns (1882) who showed that in those over the age of 50, fractures of the forearm and hip were more frequent in women than in men. Albright et al (1941) first demonstrated a clear relationship between the menopause and oestrogen deficiency, and osteoporosis. With an ageing population, post-menopausal osteoporosis now represents an enormous public health problem. It has been estimated by the National Osteoporosis Society that the cost of non-fatal hip fractures in the United Kingdom is about £180 000 000 annually. Albright (1941) first postulated that a reduction in gonadal function leads to osteoporosis and demonstrated that treatment with stilboestrol could reverse the negative calcium balance in a post-menopausal osteoporotic woman (Albright, 1941). Furthermore he recognized that osteoporosis was accompanied by thin skin and suggested that post-menopausal osteoporosis may be a disease of protein metabolism. Albright also assumed that post-menopausal osteoporosis resulted from a decrease in osteoblastic activity but Nordin et al (1981) demonstrated that in fact it is an increase in osteoblastic activity which is responsible.

The mechanism whereby diminished ovarian function leads to a decrease in osteoblast activity remains unclear. It has been suggested that oestrogen deficiency results in malabsorption of dietary calcium (Nordin, 1960). This is unlikely to be so, however, as the serum calcium concentration in post-menopausal osteoporosis is not reduced and is sometimes elevated. The concentration of parathyroid hormone is within normal limits. It has been suggested that calcitonin plays a central role in the aetiology of post-menopausal osteoporosis. This is a peptide hormone released by the para-follicular cells of the thyroid gland. Calcitonin reduces both the number and activity of osteoclastic cells. Stevenson and Whitehead (1982) showed a decrease in calcitonin levels after the menopause and concluded that oestrogen deficiency may lead to a reduced level of calcitonin and thus less inhibition of osteoclastic activity, therefore causing osteoporosis. Subsequent studies have failed to confirm this however (Chestnut, 1984; Tiegs et al, 1984).

Recently post-menopausal osteoporosis studies have mostly concentrated on calcium and calcium related hormones, ignoring the organic matrix. The latter is largely collagen and makes up approximately 35% of dry defatted bone mass. The organic matrix of bone acts rather like internal girders and confers on bone its tensile strength, and it has been suggested that it is a decline in this organic matrix that is the primary pathological event leading to osteoporosis (Brincat et al, 1987a,d). The association of thin skin, low in collagen, and osteoporosis, and thin skin with such conditions as osteogenesis imperfecta and steroid-induced osteoporosis provides some evidence for the suggestion that post-menopausal osteoporosis is also a generalized connective tissue disorder, thus confirming Albright's original impressions (Albright, 1941).

Clinical implications

As a result of osteoporosis, bones are more liable to fracture spontaneously or as a result of minimal trauma. The three most common types of fracture are distal, radial and ulnar (Colles'), vertebral body and the neck of femur. These have a combined incidence of 40% in white women over the age of 65 (Crilly et al, 1978). Colles' fractures frequently occur as a result of falls. Approximately 0.5% of women over the age of 70 will sustain this fracture each year—12 times the incidence in age-matched men (Alffram and Bauer, 1962). The crush fractures of the vertebra typically involve T8–L4 and may occur spontaneously with normal activity such as sitting up from a chair or bed. They often cause severe pain and disability, can result in a loss of up to 5 inches in height, or produce marked kyphosis (Dowager's hump). Twenty-five per cent of women over the age of 65 will have either clinical or radiological evidence of such a fracture.

Fracture of the neck of the femur is the most significant traumatic conse-quence of post-menopausal osteoporosis. The affected population tends to be older and the associated mortality and morbidity greater than with any other fracture. Approximately 27% of women who sustain such a fracture die within one year (Miller, 1978). The death rate from osteoporotic hip fractures is greater than that of carcinoma of the breast and endometrium combined. At least 20% of those injured suffer from considerable loss of mobility one year after the fracture.

A number of risk factors for the development of post-menopausal osteoporosis have been identified:

1. White (caucasian) women are at greater risk of developing osteoporosis than black women because they start off with a lesser peak bone mass and may lose bone at a faster rate.
2. Underweight women, or women with a small build, may be at a greater risk because of reduced peripheral conversion of adrenal androgens to oestrogen.
3. Anorexia leading to amenorrhoea and hyperoestrogenism leads to severe osteoporosis.
4. A sedentary life-style encourages bone loss.
5. Although exercise may have a beneficial effect on the skeleton, strenuous exercise producing amenorrhoea will lead to significant bone loss. Warren et al (1986) have shown that young ballet dancers have a high incidence of late menarche and secondary amenorrhoea resulting in an increased incidence of skeletal fractures.
6. Corticosteroid therapy causes osteoporosis, but the mechanism for this is unclear.
7. Excessive alcohol and caffeine consumption, and smoking are known to increase bone loss.
8. A high protein diet is also thought to lead to increased bone loss, indicated by an increase in calcium excretion by the kidneys.
9. Nulliparity is a risk factor. It is possible that during pregnancy some of the age-related bone losses are arrested so that a woman who has had repeated pregnancies will have a greater bone mass at the time of her menopause.

A number of prospective studies have confirmed Albright's findings that oestrogen can prevent post-menopausal osteoporosis (Lindsay et al, 1978; Christiansen et al, 1980; Natchigall et al, 1980) and epidemiological studies have shown that this will lead to a reduction in the incidence of fractures. Ross et al (1984) have estimated that five years of oestrogen replacement therapy will halve a woman's risk of developing osteoporotic fractures. Lindsay et al (1984) have suggested that 0.625 mg of conjugated equine oestrogens is sufficient for protection of the skeleton. Recent studies have shown, however, that the higher oestradiol levels achieved with a sub-cutaneous oestradiol/testosterone implant will lead to a reversal of earlier post-menopausal bone loss (Savvas et al, 1988). Figure 3. There is also some evidence that progestogens may be effective in preventing osteoporosis due to stimulation of new bone formation (Lindsay et al, 1978).

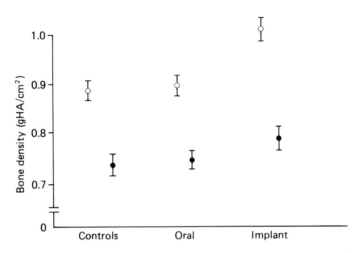

Figure 3. Mean (± SEM) spine and femoral neck bone density in post-menopausal women, untreated and on oral and implant therapy. ○ spine, ● proximal femur. Modified from Savves et al (1988).

Skin

The skin, one of the largest organs in the body, undergoes changes after the menopause. Many of these changes have formerly been attributed to the 'ageing' process but are in reality due to oestrogen deficiency. The skin of post-menopausal women who are on sex hormone replacement therapy has been shown to contain more collagen than women of the same age who are on no treatment (Brincat et al, 1983).

Skin thickness declines after the menopause in a rapid fashion at a rate very similar to the decline in bone mass. This decline cannot be explained by age alone; skin collagen declines by some 30% in the first ten years after the menopause, an amount that is comparable to bone loss over the same period (Brincat et al, 1985, 1987a,c; Figure 4).

Prospective studies on skin collagen have shown that even though collagen was lost as a result of duration of ovarian failure, it was possible to

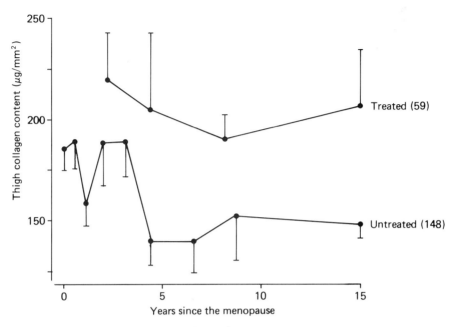

Figure 4. Thigh skin collagen content (M ± sᴇ) with years since menopause in 148 untreated post-menopausal women and in 59 post-menopausal women who had been on sex hormone treatment for between 2 and 10 years.

restore collagen to pre-menopausal levels within six months of initiating hormone replacement therapy (Brincat, 1987a,b,c,e). If hormone replacement therapy was initiated early there was no decline in the level of skin collagen or in skin thickness.

It is our belief that sex hormone deprivation after the menopause, in particular oestrogen deficiency, leads to a generalized connective tissue loss. This would therefore be the initial pathology in osteoporotic bone loss, with reduced mineral content of bone following the breakdown of the organic collagenous matrix (Brincat and Studd, 1988).

Both oestrogen and androgen receptors have been identified in the fibro-blasts of the skin (Black et al, 1970; Stumpf et al, 1976). More recently, oestrogen receptors have finally been identified on osteoblasts (Kaplan, 1987), lending weight to the argument that sex steroids have a direct action on osteoblasts. In addition, the possibility of oestrogens working on both fibroblasts and osteoblasts indirectly, through an intermediary hormone such as growth hormone must be considered (Vashinav et al, 1984).

The epidermis has not been studied extensively although oestradiol receptors do exist in its basal cell layer (Shahrad and Marks, 1977). Punnonen (1973) claimed a significantly higher mitotic activity in the epidermis in in vitro studies exposing epidermal cells to oestrogen. He also showed that the epidermis became thinner, the longer the time interval between castration and investigation in studies that he carried out on women.

Genito-urinary system

The mucosal linings of the vagina and urethra have the highest concentrations of oestrogen receptors in the body and are therefore, not surprisingly, extremely sensitive to alterations in the oestrogen levels. The trigone of the bladder, derived embryologically from the uro-genital sinus, also appears to undergo atrophic changes after the menopause.

The vaginal epithelium of post-menopausal women becomes attenuated, pale and almost transparent as a result of a decrease in vascularity. Marked atrophic changes in the vagina can result in atrophic vaginitis, with the vaginal epithelium becoming thin, inflamed and ulcerated.

The cervix, instead of protruding into the vagina, atrophies, retracts and becomes flush with the apex of the vault. The uterine corpus itself becomes smaller with a return to the 1:2 corpus:cervix ratio of childhood.

The endometrium becomes thin and atrophic, although cystic glands may persist for many years. In some women with a higher endogenous oestrogen production, the endometrium may be active and proliferative and even hyperplastic. Such women tend to be obese since after the menopause the chief source of oestrogens is derived from peripheral conversion of cholesterol in adipose tissue.

Atrophy of both the vagina and the urethra have symptomatic sequelae which can continue to be troublesome. These include dyspareunia, apareunia and recurrent bacterial infections. In the urethra, repeated infections may lead to fibrosis which predisposes to frequency, dysuria and urgency referred to as the 'urethral syndrome' (Smith, 1972). The submucosal vascular plexus of the urethra contribute to sphincteric function and are oestrogen dependent (Versi and Cardozo, 1985), as may be the collagen content of the urethral submucosal connective tissue (Versi et al, 1988). Oestrogen receptors have been detected in the human female urethra (Iosif et al, 1981), suggesting a direct action of the hormone. It would appear, therefore, that both the genital and the lower urinary tract are influenced by oestrogens.

Incontinence

Osborne (1976) studied 600 women aged between 35 and 60 and was unable to show an increased prevalence of incontinence at the time of the menopause. Iosif and Bekassy (1984) on the other hand in a survey of 902 Swedish women aged 61 found a 29.2% incidence of urinary incontinence. The debate as to whether ovarian failure leads to incontinence still rages.

Versi (1986) reported a high incidence of stress incontinence, frequency, nocturia and urgency in peri- and post-menopausal women. Stanton et al (1983) found the incidence of pain on micturition in a similar group of women to be 30%.

Tables 3 and 4 (Versi, 1986) indicate symptomatology elicited by history alone, and urodynamically proven diagnoses, respectively. (There was no pre-menopausal control group for comparison.) These results suggest that urological changes occur in the climacteric. As in the case of bone loss, analyses relying upon a sharp definition of the menopause may be unreliable

Table 3. A comparison of lower urinary symptomatology in peri- and post-menopausal women.

	Peri-menopausal 54* 46.5 ± 0.6†	Post-menopausal 89* 52.2 ± 0.5†
Stress incontinence		
occasional	33.3%	40.4%
frequent	9.3%	10.1%
Frequency (>8 per day)	31.5%	28.2%
Nocturia (>once per night)	29.6%	29.2%
Urgency		
occasional	16.7%	33.7%
frequent	31.5%	21.3%
Painful micturition	13.0%	10.3%
Poor stream	5.6%	10.1%
Incomplete bladder emptying	11.3%	13.0%

* Number of women studied. † Mean age ± SD.

Table 4. The prevalence of urodynamically diagnosed pathology in women undergoing the climacteric.

	Peri-menopausal	Post-menopausal
Total	54	89
Normals	33 (61%)	62 (70%)
Genuine stress incontinence	10 (19%)	12 (13%)
Detrusor instability	5 (10%)	10 (11%)
Voiding difficulty	3 (6%)	4 (4%)
Urethral syndrome	0 (0%)	1 (1%)

since they do not make any allowance for the possibility of fluctuating to low oestrogen levels affecting urinary function some time prior to the menopause. One third of the population looked at by Versi (1986) had abnormal urodynamic results. Genuine stress incontinence, detrusor instability, and voiding difficulties were the most commonly found abnormalities.

Urethral pressure profilometry revealed that post-menopausal women had weaker urethral sphincters under stress than the peri-menopausal groups (Versi, 1986). A later study by the same group demonstrated a correlation between urethral pressure measurements and skin collagen content (Versi et al, 1988). Increases in urethral pressure have been noted after hormone replacement therapy (Faber and Heidenreich, 1977; Walter et al, 1978; Hilton and Stanton, 1983). Since increases in skin collagen with hormone replacement therapy have also been noted (Brincat et al, 1987b,e) it is suggested that the beneficial effects on urethral function may be mediated by beneficial effects on collagen control (Versi et al, 1988).

In summary, therefore, lower urinary tract problems are seemingly increased as a result of oestrogen deficiency after the menopause. It is still not clear, however, what the effects of increasing age are on urinary tract function. Likewise it is still not clear which symptoms are specifically due to oestrogen deficiency, although a large number of women attending a menopause clinic will complain of such symptoms and claim benefit with oestrogen therapy.

INVESTIGATIONS AND DIAGNOSIS

With increasing awareness, it is no longer just the women with the short-term symptoms of the menopause who are presenting to specialist clinics. Increasingly women are demanding prophylaxis for the long-term consequences of the menopause even though, at presentation they may be apparently asymptomatic.

Misdiagnosis is unlikely in the women who present with the characteristic picture of acute vasomotor disturbances and symptoms of lower genital tract atrophy coupled with oligo- or amenorrhoea. Other conditions associated with flushing and sweating such as phaeochromocytoma, carcinoid disease and thyroid disease cause additional symptoms and should make the diagnosis obvious.

Plasma gonadotrophins and oestrogen concentrations fluctuate widely during the climacteric (Chakravarti et al, 1976) and detailed biochemical investigations are often of little value in diagnosis, with symptoms always being the best guide. In premature menopause, or when there is some additional doubt as to whether the menopause has occurred or not, such as in hysterectomized women, a high serum FSH should be sufficient to establish the diagnosis. It might also be useful to estimate serum oestradiol levels. Endocrine assessments cannot accurately predict the eventual severity and duration of symptoms nor the response to therapy.

Similarly, the intensity of short-term symptoms of the menopause bear no relationship to the severity of the long-term consequences. Methods for assessing bone mass accurately such as bone densitometry or quantitative computed tomography (QCT) analysis are cumbersome and have no place as routine screening tools.

It is crucial to establish whether psychological disturbances that a patient may be presenting with are due to oestrogen deficiency or result from coincidental but current social, domestic or economic crises. When diagnosis proves difficult, biochemical investigations may be of value because high plasma oestrogen levels exclude ovarian failure although the converse does not necessarily apply. With the latter, it has been our practice to give the patient the benefit of the doubt and embark on a course of hormone replacement therapy.

Climacteric depression responds rapidly and well to hormone replacement especially to implant therapy (Montgomery et al, 1987) and therefore if, despite this therapy, the woman still has not responded, then one can assume that the woman's psychological symptoms are not due to sex hormone imbalance or deficiency and she would probably be better helped by the psychiatrists.

TREATMENT

The treatment of choice for the management of menopausal symptoms and sequelae is oestrogen therapy which should in most cases successfully correct this multi-system deficiency state. Other treatments available only serve, at best, to manage a particular symptom without striking at the root of the problem. In some cases serious side-effects occur that could be worse than any possible from properly managed hormone replacement.

Therapy is divided into non-hormonal and hormonal.

Non-hormonal

Geist and Mintz (1937) proposed irradiating the pituitary so as to suppress excess production of gonadotrophins which they believed caused flushing. Their results were not encouraging. More recently, suppression of pituitary activity using LHRH analogues has proved not only to be useless in suppressing flushes but actually to provoke such flushes (Lightman et al, 1982).

Vitamin E has been proposed for the treatment and the prevention of many sex-related problems but apart from one study (McLaren, 1949) this has never been substantiated.

Sedatives and tranquillizers have been widely prescribed for over a century with barbiturates, diazepam and similar drugs. Such therapy only adds to the lethargy and general loss of interest in life and certainly does nothing to prevent symptoms like flushing, although surprisingly they have been prescribed for this symptom as well. It is a sad fact of contemporary life that about 40% of middle-aged and elderly women have had long courses of psychoactive drugs. At last, however, an editorial in the *Lancet* asks the question 'Must we poison our old patients?' (Editorial, 1988).

Amongst the adrenergic agents currently used, clonidine, an α-adrenergic agonist seems to have some potential. Clayden et al (1974) supervised a multi-centre, placebo controlled, cross-over study on 100 women and reported significant benefit in controlling the severity and duration of flushes with minimal side-effects. It is noted that in common with many similar studies, there was no difference in menopause symptoms until the therapy was crossed-over. Lindsay and Hart (1978) failed, however, to find any difference in flushing episodes when clonidine was compared to placebo.

Propranolol has been tried with conflicting results. Alcoff et al (1981) obtained a difference in flushing episodes when compared to placebo. Methyldopa (Tulandi et al, 1984) and naproxen (Haataja et al, 1984) have also been suggested but once more results as regards their use in the relief of flushes are conflicting. Ethamsylate, used principally in the treatment of menorrhagia, has been tried and Harrison (1981) reported some good results.

Hormonal

Progestogens

Progestogens can suppress flushes (Appleby, 1962; Patterson, 1982); both norethisterone (Patterson, 1982) and medroxyprogesterone have been reported as useful (Schiff et al, 1980). Progestogens have been shown to be useful in the prevention of post-menopausal bone loss and several studies have shown this. The gestogens used in these studies were medroxy-progesterone, megestrol and norethisterone (Lindsay et al, 1978; Lobo et al, 1984).

Anabolic steroids

In women, androgens have been used in the prevention and treatment of post-menopausal osteoporosis. Stanozolol, an anabolic steroid, has been studied extensively and shown to increase total body calcium in patients with established osteoporosis (Chestnut et al, 1979; Chestnut, 1984); its use in the prevention of post-menopausal bone loss, however remains to be determined.

Oestrogens

Oestrogen replacement therapy is the appropriate overall treatment for problems caused by ovarian failure. The aim of a therapeutic regimen is to provide the most effective treatment with the least side-effects. Oestrogens may be given either orally or parenterally—percutaneously, trans-vaginally, as cream or more recently as skin patches. Oestrogens can also be given subcutaneously as implants. The pharmacodynamics and biochemical effects of exogenous oestrogens can vary markedly with the route of administration.

Oral oestrogens. The oral route is the most popular (Judd et al, 1981). Its major difference from the parenteral route is that administered oestrogens are exposed to the gastrointestinal tract, the portal venous system and the liver. Oestradiol is preferentially converted to oestrone in the gastrointestinal tract (Ryan and Engel, 1953). The portal venous system rapidly transfers the absorbed steroid, almost in the form of a 'bolus' into hepatic tissue where much of the administered oestrogen is metabolized and inactivated before the systemic circulation is reached. This is known as the 'first-pass' effect.

Glucuronidation of oestrogen occurs almost exclusively in the liver, so percutaneous and subcutaneous oestradiol administration are not associated with an increase in plasma oestrone-3-glucuronide levels (Campbell and Whitehead, 1982).

Because of the first-pass effect, oral oestrogens have to be given at a higher dose than parenteral therapy to maintain relief of symptoms. Induction of liver enzymes, particularly the glucoronidase enzymes, by other drugs such as anti-epileptics may result in such a rapid oestrogen inactivation that the administered steroid is not clinically effective. Also, oral oestrogens may influence the production of renin substrate, anti-thrombin III, and high and low density lipoproteins.

Oral oestrogens are more potent than parenterally administered oestrogens in elevating HDL-cholesterol (Brenner et al, 1982) thereby increasing the HDL/LDL ratio with the consequent beneficial implications for arterial disease (Gordon et al, 1977).

By depressing anti-thrombin III activity, oral oestrogens might be contraindicated in women with a history of clotting disorder (Van der Meer et al, 1973), and likewise in hypertensives due to the theoretical risk of alteration of renin substrate (Laragh et al, 1967). It must be emphasized, however, that these last two contraindications and other theoretical ones generally refer to synthetic oral oestrogens and therefore should not be extrapolated for the natural oral oestrogens that are used in hormone replacement.

By virtue of their structure, the synthetic oestrogens have a greater affinity for the oestrogen receptor and are not substrates for the intracellular enzymes which normally downgrade oestrogens (Brenner et al, 1982). This leads to an enhanced hepatic potency and because of this, synthetic oestrogens should be avoided in post-menopausal women unless given in small doses.

Parenteral oestrogens. Parenteral oestrogens are particularly advantageous when oral therapy causes epigastric discomfort and flatulence, and when patients have a psychological aversion to taking tablets. They have all the beneficial effects of oral oestrogens.

Vaginal oestrogen creams. These have long been used in the treatment of atrophic vaginitis, on the assumption that they produced a local effect only. Whitehead et al (1978) however showed that the plasma levels of oestrone and oestradiol achieved using a standard regimen daily dose of 1.25 mg of conjugated oestrogen cream are the same or higher than those produced by the same dose of oral conjugated oestrogens.

Very low doses of vaginal oestrogens (0.1 mg) daily are capable of producing significant changes in vaginal cytology and do not cause a rise in plasma oestrogens (Dyer et al, 1982). At this low serum level, however, there is no relief of the generalized symptoms of the climacteric and there are as yet no long-term studies indicating that even this low dosage does not cause deleterious effects on the endometrium when given continuously for a long time. Preparations such as oestriol are available.

The rate of absorption of oestrogens from the vagina depend on the state of the vagina. As vascularity decreases, so does absorption. The rate of absorption also depends on the medium in which the oestradiol is suspended (Schiff et al, 1977).

Percutaneous oestrogen creams. This mode of delivery is becoming increasingly popular. A preparation which involves the daily application of oestradiol gel on the skin (Besins) is available. The standard manufacturer's recommended dose is 5 g cream containing 3 mg of oestradiol daily. The method of administration gives a physiological serum oestradiol to oestrone ratio by bypassing the enterohepatic circulation. The avoidance of the first-pass liver effect is common to both percutaneous and subcutaneous therapy.

Various studies have shown that this method gives good relief of symptoms and is safe in post-menopausal women (Sitruk-Ware et al, 1980; Strecker et al, 1980; Brincat et al, 1984a), in whom it has also been shown to increase skin collagen content, at the same dosage (Brincat et al, 1987e).

The daily application of cream (gel) requires patient compliance since some women find it sticky. The gel dries up quickly, however, and our own experience has not shown any real problems. Percutaneous cream leads to a relatively higher increase in serum oestradiol and achieves serum levels that are maintained for longer when compared to oral preparations (Sitruk-Ware et al, 1980; Lyrenas et al, 1981).

The transdermal patch has been recently developed and can administer oestradiol at controlled rates of 0.025, 0.5, and 0.1 mg/day, depending on the surface area of the patch. Steady concentrations can be obtained if the systems are worn for 72 hours and changed twice weekly (Vickers, 1980).

Utian (1987) showed that the Estraderm patches currently used are as efficacious as Premarin in the relief of symptoms of the climacteric and like Premarin need to have an added progestogen if endometrial hyperplasia is to be avoided (see below). The area of application of both percutaneous and transdermal systems should be changed regularly because of the possibility of itching and skin irritation.

Subcutaneous implants. Subcutaneous implants have been used to treat the climacteric syndrome for almost 40 years (Greenblatt and Buran, 1949). The technique of insertion is simple and can be done in an outpatients clinic under local anaesthesia. Gonadotrophin levels fall dramatically within two weeks of implantation and do not return to pre-treatment levels before six months if a 100 mg oestradiol implant is used (Thom et al, 1981). Oestradiol levels similarly rise to reach a peak at two to three months and are back to pre-treatment levels by six months.

The use of subcutaneous hormone implants avoids the need for daily patient compliance. Furthermore, a testosterone pellet (100 mg) can be safely inserted and thus give the patient further relief of the symptoms of lethargy and loss of libido (Studd et al, 1977; Montgomery et al, unpublished data). Methyltestosterone (which might be useful for the treatment of psychosexual symptoms) is hepatotoxic when administered orally.

Implants give good symptomatic relief for up to six months (Brincat et al, 1984b), have few side-effects and complications are rare (Cardozo et al, 1984). Even more interesting is the apparent increase in bone mass that is possible in post-menopausal women using oestradiol implant regimes. In a recent study, Savvas et al (1988) showed that a population of women who had been on oestradiol and testosterone implants for between two and ten years had a higher bone mass than a comparable group who had been on oral therapy, who in turn had a bone mass as high as a population of very early post-menopausal women. Furthermore, a prospective study now underway by the same authors is showing a considerable increase in bone mass occurring in women on oestradiol-only implants. A 5% increase in vertebral bone density was found after six months and a 9% increase after one year. The increase in the proximal femoral bone density was only about 40% of the spine increase because the trabecular bone of the femur is less bio-logically active.

The conclusion from this and other studies is that although it is possible to maintain bone mass using oral preparations, the higher oestradiol levels achieved with a subcutaneous oestradiol/testosterone implant will lead to a gain in bone mass and a reversal in bone loss. Similar results are obtained when collagen content and thickness of skin is studied when women receive oestradiol implants (Brincat et al, 1987b,c).

Oral preparations currently used can only increase bone mass in early post-menopausal women if they are combined with pharmacological doses of an anti-resorptive agent such as calcitonin (Meschia et al, 1988). This would entail at least two injections a week.

Campbell and Whitehead (1977) showed significant relief of climacteric symptoms using the most widely used dose and preparation, 1.25 mg of conjugated oestrogens daily. Most current regimens are given continuously as opposed to having one pill-free week every four and opposed with a fixed period of gestogens.

Alternative forms of therapy which avoid the first-pass effect on the liver are simple to use, are efficacious and have a high patient acceptability.

The importance of clinical opposed therapy

It has been established that if oestrogens are given on their own and continuously, the incidence of endometrial hyperplasia and the possibility of causing a well differentiated adenocarcinoma of the endometrium is increased, whichever route of administration is used. Assessment of oestrogen concentration within the nuclei of endometrial cells has shown a higher level of oestradiol than oestrone (Whitehead et al, 1981), so it is likely that oestradiol has a greater effect on cell proliferation.

Oral oestrogen may be associated with a lower incidence of endometrial hyperplasia than other methods. If, in exceptional circumstances, oestrogens need to be used alone then it would be safer to use such preparations cyclically (i.e. 21 days out of every 28). The addition of cyclical progestogen therapy for 13 days each month has been shown to abolish initially the risk of endometrial hyperplasia (Table 4; Studd et al, 1980; Studd and Thom, 1981; Studd and Magos, 1988).

In women who do not want cyclical bleeding or who would be better managed without a monthly withdrawal bleed, it is possible to start continuous regimens of oral oestrogens and combine this with continuous progestogens. By adjusting the progestogen dose appropriately, it is possible to obtain 100% amenorrhoea within 6–9 months of therapy (Magos et al, 1985). No endometrial hyperplasia occurred in one study where women were followed up for over two years (Magos et al, 1986; Studd and Magos, 1988).

There is no evidence, however that any extra benefit or protection anywhere is achieved if gestogens are prescribed in the absence of a uterus (Studd et al, 1986). Indeed the protective effect of oestrogens on the cardiovascular system might be compromised by gestogens (Lobo et al, 1987). The protective effect of gestogens against breast cancer is extremely controversial (Miller and Anderson, 1988). Evidence in favour is weak and certainly there is no consensus (Lobo et al, 1987). Gambrell (1986, 1988) has suggested that such a protective effect does exist but should be considered in conjunction with the evidence of Pike et al (1983) on progestogens increasing the incidence of breast cancer. Other authors have not shown any difference in the incidence of breast cancer when women on oestrogens alone were compared to those on combined preparations (Hunt et al, 1987).

Contraindications to hormone replacement therapy

As with all treatment, oestrogen therapy requires consideration of the severity of the illness to be treated and the possible side-effects. Most workers would accept that breast carcinoma and endometrial carcinoma are contraindications, but scientific support for these objections is hard to find. It is not unusual that women with oestrogen-dependent tumours are prepared to take the risk of oestrogen therapy because their lives are made so unbearable by menopausal symptoms. There is in fact no evidence that oestrogen therapy produces a recurrence of breast or endometrial carcinoma but if a recurrence does occur it is likely that oestrogens will be blamed.

Hypertension, varicose veins, a previous thrombotic episode, diabetes, endometriosis and fibroids are classically regarded as contraindications, but once again, there is little evidence that this is so. There is no evidence that natural oestrogens (i.e. oestradiol, oestrone or oestriol) cause any elevation of blood pressure in normotensive or hypertensive women (Hammond et al, 1979). Natural progesterone taken orally seems to lower blood pressure in established hypertensives (Rylance et al, 1985) in contradiction to previous belief. There is no evidence that oestrogens either affect coagulation, fibrolysis and platelet behaviour, or cause deep vein thrombosis (Boston Collaborative Drug Surveillance Programme, 1974; Studd et al, 1978; Thom et al, 1978).

The avoidance of the first-pass liver effect by utilizing percutaneous or subcutaneous routes give even less reason to suppose that synthesis of coagulation factors from the liver should be stimulated. Although synthetic ethinyloestradiol and mestranol are diabetogenic, the natural oestrogens are not (Thom et al, 1977; Studd et al, 1978).

Endometriosis and fibroids are certainly responsive to endogenous and exogenous oestrogens and it is possible that such therapy will stimulate activity of these benign gynaecological conditions. This does not in practice represent any clinical problem because treatment can easily be discontinued. Patients who have undergone a hysterectomy with or without oophorectomy for these conditions do not have any contraindications for oestrogen therapy. This is particularly true for endometriosis when the woman may be quite young and may have suffered a surgical castration for her condition.

CONCLUSION

The changes that occur with changing ovarian function culminating with the menopause cause profound changes to a woman. Although not all women have the distressing short-term symptoms, there is no doubt that all experience an endocrinological deficiency syndrome leading to multi-system problems, ranging from connective tissue loss to psychological disturbances.

The hormone deficiency state of menopausal women must be recognized. With increasing longevity of the population and the increase in morbidity and eventual mortality as a result of sex hormone deficiency, the philosophy of whom to treat and who not to treat deserves reappraisal. There is a poor correlation between the short-term symptoms and the long-term consequences of the menopause and therefore it is not possible to select women for treatment on the basis of their immediate symptomatology alone. A case can be made for the widespread use of sex hormone replacement so as to improve the quality of life and not just its quantity (Whitehead and Studd, 1988).

With continuing developments, sex hormone replacement is becoming increasingly safe and its benefits are seemingly even more extensive than once supposed, especially in the prophylaxis of cardiovascular disease and osteoporosis. Depriving a woman of hormone replacement for spurious or theoretical reasons should be considered very carefully since very often there are no real contraindications.

REFERENCES

Alcoff JM, Campbell D, Tribble D, Oldfield B & Cruess O (1981) Double blind, placebo controlled crossover trial of Propranolol as treatment for menopausal vasomotor symptoms. *Clinical Therapeutics* 3: 356–364.

Alffram PS & Bauer G (1962) Epidemiology of fractures of the forearm. *Journal of Bone and Joint Surgery* 44A: 105–104.

Allbright F, Smith PH & Richardson AM (1941) Postmenopausal osteoporosis—its clinical features. *Journal of the American Medical Association* 116: 2465–2474.

Amudsen DW & Diers CJ (1973) The age of the menopause in medieval Europe. *Human Biology* 45: 605–608.

Appleby B (1962) Norethisterone in the control of menopausal symptoms. *Lancet* i: 407–409.

Aylward M (1975) Oestrogens, plasma, tryptophan levels in peri-menopausal patients. In Campbell S (ed.) *The management of the menopause and postmenopausal years*, pp 135–147. London: University Parthenon Press.

Baker TG (1963) A Quantitative and Cytological Study of Germ Cells in Human Ovaries. *Proceedings of the Royal Society of London, Series B* 158: 417–433.

Ballinger CB (1975) Psychiatric morbidity and the menopause. Screening of the general population sample. *British Medical Journal* 3: 344–346.

Ballinger CB (1977) Psychiatric morbidity and the menopause. Survey of gynaecological outpatient clinic. *British Journal of Psychiatry* 131: 83–89.

Black NM, Shuster S & Bottoms E (1970) Osteoporosis, Skin collagen and androgen. *British Medical Journal* 4: 773–774.

Boston Collaborative Drug Surveillance Programme (1974) Surgically confirmed gall bladder venous thrombo embolism and breast tumours in relation to postmenopausal oestrogen therapy. *New England Journal of Medicine* 290: 15–19.

Brenner PM, MashChak CA, Cobo RA et al (1982) Potency and hepato-cellular effects of oestrogen after oral, percutaneous, subcutaneous administration. In Van Keep PA, Utian W & Vermular A (eds) *The Controversial Climacteric*, pp 103–125. Lancaster: MTP Press.

Brincat M & Studd JWW (1988) Skin and the menopause. *The Menopause* 8: 85–101.

Brincat M, Moniz CE, Studd JWW et al (1983) Sex hormones and skin collagen content in postmenopausal women. *British Medical Journal* 287: 1337–1338.

Brincat TM, deTrafford JC, Lafferty K, Roberts VC & Studd JW (1984a) A role for oestrogen in peripheral vasomotor control and menopausal flushing—a preliminary report. *British Journal of Obstetrics and Gynaecology* 11: 1107–1110.

Brincat M, Magos AL, Studd JWW et al (1984b) Subcutaneous hormone implants for the control of climacteric symptoms:—A prospective study. *Lancet* **i:** 16–18.

Brincat M, Moniz CJ, Studd JWW et al (1985) Long term effects of the menopause and sex hormones on skin thickness. *British Journal of Obstetrics and Gynaecology* **92:** 256–259.

Brincat M, Moniz CF, Kabalan S et al (1987a) Decline in skin collagen content and metacarpal index after the menopause and its prevention with sex hormone replacement. *British Journal of Obstetrics and Gynaecology* **94:** 126–129.

Brincat M, Versi E, Studd JWW et al (1987b) Skin collagen changes in postmenopausal women receiving different regimes of oestrogen therapy. *Obstetrics and Gynecology* **70:** 123–127.

Brincat M, Wong A, Studd JWW et al (1987c) The response of skin thickness and metacarpal index to oestradiol therapy in postmenopausal women. *Obstetrics and Gynecology* **70:** 538–541.

Brincat M, Kabalan S, Studd JWW et al (1987d) A study of the relationship of skin collagen content, skin thickness and bone mass in the postmenopausal woman. *Obstetrics and Gynecology* **70:** 840–845.

Brincat M, Moniz CF, Kabalan S et al (1987e) Skin collagen changes in postmenopausal women treated with oestradiol gel. *Maturitas* **9:** 1–5.

Bruns P (1882) Die Allgemaine Lebra von der Knochenbruchen. *Deutshe Chirvrgie* **27:** 1–400.

Bush TL, Barnett-Connor E, Cowan LD et al (1987) Cardiovascular mortality and non-contraceptive use of oestrogen in women: results from the Lipid Research Clinic's Programme follow-up study. *Circulation* **75:** 1102.

Campbell S (1975) Psychometric studies on the effect of natural oestrogens in postmenopausal women. In Campbell S (ed.) *Management of the menopause and postmenopausal years*, pp 149–158. Lancaster: MTP Press.

Campbell S & Whitehead MI (1977) Oestrogen therapy and the menopausal syndrome. *Clinics in Obstetrics and Gynaecology* **4** (supplement 1): 31–47.

Campbell S & Whitehead MI (1982) Potency and hepato-cellular effects of oestrogens after oral, percutaneous and subcutaneous administration. In Van Keep PA, Utian W & Vermeulen A (eds) *The Controversial Climacteric*, pp 103–125. Lancaster: MTP Press.

Cardozo L, Gibb D, Studd JWW, Tuck S, Thom M & Cooper D (1984) The use of hormone implants for the climacteric symptoms. *American Journal of Obstetrics and Gynecology* **1:** 336–337.

Chakravati S, Collins WP, Forecart JD et al (1976) Hormonal profiles after the menopause. *British Medical Journal* **2:** 784–786.

Chestnut CH (1984) Synthetic salmon calcitonin, diphosphales and anabolic steroids in the treatment of postmenopausal osteoporosis. *Osteoporosis*. Proceedings of the Copenhagen International Symposium on Osteoporosis Vol 2, pp 549–555.

Chestnut CH III, Ivey JL, Nelp WB et al (1979) Assessment of anabolic steroids and calcitonin in the treatment of osteoporosis. In Barzel US (ed.) *Osteoporosis II*, pp 135–150. New York: Grune and Stratton.

Christiansen C, Christiansen MS, McNain P, Hagen C, Stockland K & Transolol I (1980) Prevention of early menopausal bone loss: controlled 2-year study in 315 normal females. *European Journal of Clinical Investigation* **10:** 273–279.

Clayden JR, Bell JW & Pollard P (1974) Menopausal flushing: double blind trial of a non-hormonal preparation. *British Medical Journal* **1:** 409–412.

Crilly RG, Horsman A, Marshall DH & Nordin BEC (1978) Bone mass in postmenopausal women after withdrawal of oestrogen/gestogen replacement therapy. *Lancet* **i:** 459–461.

Crook D, Godsland IF & Wynn V (1988) Ovarian hormones and plasma lipoproteins. *The Menopause* **15:** 168–180.

De Fazio J, Meldrum DR, Winer JH & Judd HC (1984) Direct action of androgens on hot flushes in a human male. *Maturitas* **6:** 3–8.

Dennerstein L & Burrows G (1978) A review of studies of the psychological symptoms found at the menopause. *Maturitas* **1:** 55–64.

Dyer G, Townsend PT, Jehowitsz J, Young O & Whitehead MI (1982) Dose related changes in vaginal cytology after topical conjugated equine oestrogens. *British Medical Journal* **284:** 789–790.

Editorial (1988) Need we poison the elderly so often? *Lancet* **ii:** 20.

Erlik Y, Tatayn IV, Meldrum DR et al (1981) Association of wakening episodes with menopausal hot flushes. *Journal of the American Medical Association* **245:** 1741–1744.

Faber P & Heidenreich J (1977) Treatment of stress incontinence with oestrogen in post-menopausal women. *Urologia Internationalis* **32:** 221–223.

Fieldman JM, Postlethwaite RW & Glenn JF (1976) Hot flushes and sweats in men with testicular insufficiency. *Archives of Internal Medicine* **136:** 606–608.

Frere G (1971) Mean age at menopause and menache in South Africa. *South African Journal of Medical Science* **36:** 21–25.

Frie JF (1980) Ageing, natural death and the compression of morbidity. *New England Journal of Medicine* **303:** 130–135.

Gambrell D (1986) Hormonal replacement therapy and breast cancer. In Greenblatt RB (ed.) *A modern approach to the perimenopausal years,* pp 176–188. Berlin, New York: Walter de Gruyrer.

Gambrell RD (1988) Studies of endometrial and breast disease with hormone replacement therapy. *The Menopause* **22:** 247–261.

Geist SH & Mintz M (1937) Pituitary radiation for the relief of menopause symptoms. *American Journal of Obstetrics and Gynecology* **33:** 643–645.

Gordan GS (1984) Prevention of bone loss and fractures in women. *Maturitas* **6:** 225–242.

Gordon T, Castelli WP, Hjorteand MC, Kannel WO & Dauber TR (1977) High density lipoprotein as a protective factor against coronary heart disease. The Framingham Study. *American Journal of Medicine* **62:** 707–714.

Greenblatt RB & Buran RR (1949) Indications for hormone pellets in the therapy of endocrine and gynaecological disorders. *American Journal of Obstetrics and Gynecology* **47:** 294–301.

Haataja M, Paul R, Gronroos M et al (1984) *Maturitas* **5:** 263–269.

Hammond CB, Jelovsek FR, Lee KC, Creasman WT & Parker RJ (1979) Effects of long term estrogen replacement therapy. 1. Metabolic effects. *American Journal of Obstetrics and Gynecology* **133:** 525–535.

Harrison RF (1981) Ethamsylate in the treatment of climacteric flushing. *Maturitas* **3:** 31–37.

Hendy MS & Burge RS (1983) Climacteric flushing in a man. *British Medical Journal* **287:** 423.

Hilton P & Stanton SL (1983) The use of intravaginal oestrogen cream in genuine stress incontinence with oestrogen in postmenopausal women. *Urologia Internationalis* **32:** 221–223.

Hunt K, Vessey M, McPherson K et al (1987) Long term surveillance of mortality and cancer incidence in women receiving hormone replacement therapy. *British Journal of Obstetrics and Gynaecology* **94:** 620–626.

Iosif CS & Bekassy Z (1984) Prevalence of genito-urinary symptoms in the late menopause. *Acta Obstetricia et Gynecologica Scandinavica* **63:** 257–260.

Iosif CS, Batia S, Ek A & Astedt B (1981) Estrogen receptors in the human female lower urinary tract. *American Journal of Obstetrics and Gynecology* **141:** 817–820.

Jazsman L (1973) Epidemiology of the climacteric complaints. *Frontiers of Hormone Research* **2:** 220–234.

Judd HL, Cleary RE, Creasman WT et al (1981) Estrogen replacement therapy. *Obstetrics and Gynecology* **58:** 267–275.

Kaplan JA (1987) Identification of oestrogen receptors on osteoblast. International Conference on Osteoporosis, Aalburg, (unpublished abstract).

Laragh JH, Sealey JE, Ledingham JG & Newton MA (1967) Oral contraceptives; Renin Aedosterone and high blood pressure. *Journal of the American Medical Association* **201:** 218–222.

Lightman SL, Jacobs AS & Maguire AK (1982) Down regulation of gonadotrophic secretion in post-menopausal women by a superactive LHRH analogue: Lack of effect on menopausal flushing. *British Journal of Obstetrics and Gynaecology* **89:** 977–980.

Lindsay R & Hart DM (1978) Failure of response of menopausal vasomotor symptoms of clonidine. *Maturitas* **1:** 21–25.

Lindsay R, Hart DH, Purdie D, Ferguson M & Clark AS (1978) Comparative effects of oestrogen and a progestagen on bone loss in postmenopausal women. *Clinical Science and Molecular Medicine* **54:** 193–198.

Lindsay R, Hart DH & Clark AS (1984) The minimum effect of oestrogen for the prevention of postmenopausal bone loss. *Obstetrics and Gynecology* **63:** 759–762.

Lobo RA, McCormick W, Singer F et al (1984) Depo-Medroxyprogesterone acetate compared with conjugated oestrogens for the treatment of post-menopausal women. *Obstetrics and Gynecology* **63**: 1–5.

Lobo RA, Wren B, Crona N et al (1987) Effects of oestrogens and progestogens on the cardiovascular system in postmenopausal women. In Zichella L, Whitehead M & van Keep PA (eds) *The Climacteric and Beyond*, pp 95–107. New Jersey: The Parthenon Publishing Group.

Lyrenas S, Carlstom K, Backstrom T & van Schoultz B (1981) A comparison of serum estrogen levels after percutaneous and oral administration of estradiol 17Beta. *British Journal of Obstetrics and Gynaecology* **83**: 181–187.

McKinlay SM & Jeffreys M (1974) The menopausal syndrome. *British Journal of Preventative and Social Medicine* **2**: 108–115.

McKinlay SM, Jeffreys K & Thompson B (1972) An investigation of the age at the menopause. *Journal of Biosocial Science* **4**: 161–166.

McLaren HC (1949) Vitamin E in the menopause. *British Medical Journal* **2**: 1378–1382.

Magos AL, Brincat M, Studd JWW et al (1985) Amenorrhoea and endometrial atrophy with continuous oral oestrogen and progestogen therapy in postmenopausal women. *Obstetrics and Gynecology* **65**: 496–499.

Magos AL, Brewster E, Singh R, O'Dowd T, Brincat M & Studd JWW (1986) The effects of norethisterone in postmenopausal women on oestrogen replacement therapy: A model for the premenstrual syndrome. *British Journal of Obstetrics and Gynaecology* **93**: 1290–1296.

Meschia M, Brincat M, Barbacini P & Crosignani PG (1988) A pilot study comparing the use of conjugated oestrogens and calcitonin to calcitonin alone in the prevention and treatment of postmenopausal osteoporosis. *European Journal of Gynaecological Endocrinology* (in press).

Miller CW (1978) Survival and ambulation following hip fractures. *Bone and Joint Surgery* **60A**: 930–934.

Miller WR & Anderson TJ (1988) Oestrogens, Progestogens and the Breast. *The Menopause* **21**: 234–246.

Montgomery JC, Appleby L, Brincat M et al (1987) Effect of oestrogen and testosterone implants on psychological disorders of the climacteric. *Lancet* **i**: 297–299.

Natchigall LE, Natchigall RH, Natchigall RD & Bechman E (1980) Estrogen replacement therapy: a 10 year prospective study in the response to osteoporosis. *Obstetrics and Gynecology* **53**: 277–281.

Neugarten BC & Kraines RJ (1965) 'Menopausal symptoms' in women of various ages. *Psychosomatic Medicine* **27**: 270–284.

Nocke W (1986) Some aspects of oogenesis, follicular growth and endocrine involution. In Greenblatt RB (ed.) *A modern approach to the perimenopausal years*, pp 11–38. Berlin, New York: Walter de Gruyter.

Nordin BEC (1960) Osteomalacia, osteoporosis and calcium deficiency. *Clinical Orthopaedics and Related Research* **17**: 235–258.

Nordin BEC, Aaron J, Speed R & Crilly RG (1981) Bone formation and resorption as the determinants of trabecular bone volume in postmenopausal osteoporosis. *Lancet* **ii**: 277–295.

Osborne JC (1976) Postmenopausal changes in micturition habits and in urine flow and urethral pressure studies. In Campbell S (ed.) *The Management of the Menopause and Post Menopausal Years*, pp 285–289. Lancaster: MTP Press.

Patterson MEL (1982) A randomized double-blind cross-over trial into the effect of norethisterone on climacteric symptoms and biochemical profiles. *British Journal of Obstetrics and Gynaecology* **89**: 464–472.

Pike HC, Henderson BE, Krailo MD, Duke A & Roy S (1983) Breast cancer in young women and use of oral contraceptives: possible modifying effect of formulation and age of use. *Lancet* **ii**: 926–929.

Punnonen R (1973) Effect of castration and peroral therapy on the skin. *Acta Obstetrica et Gynaecologica Scandinavica* **21** (supplement): 1–44.

Ross RK, Paganini-Hill A, Mack TN et al (1981) Menopausal estrogen therapy and protection from death from ischeamic heart disease. *Lancet* **i**: 858–861.

Ross RK, Paganini-Hill A & Mack JM (1984) Reduction in fractures and other effects of estrogen replacement therapy in human population. *Osteoporosis*. Proceedings of the Copenhagen International Symposium on Osteoporosis **1**: 289–297.

Ryan KJ & Engel LL (1953) The interconversion of oestrone and estradiol by human tissue slices. *Endocrinology* **52**: 287–291.

Rylance PB, Brincat M, Lafferty K et al (1985) Natural progesterone and antihypertensive action. *British Medical Journal* **290**: 13–14.

Sarrel PM (1988) Sexuality. *The Menopause* **6**: 65–75.

Savvas M, Studd JWW, Fogelman I, Dooley M, Montgomery J & Murby B (1988) Skeletal effects of oral oestrogen compared with subcutaneous oestrogen and testosterone in postmenopausal women. *British Journal of Medicine* **297**: 331–333.

Schiff I, Tulchinsky D & Ryan KJ (1977) Vaginal absorption of estrone and 17B Oestradiol. *Fertility and Sterility* **28**: 1063–1065.

Schiff I, Tulchinsky D, Cramer D & Ryan KJ (1980) Oral medroxyprogesterone in treatment of postmenopausal symptoms. *Journal of the American Medical Association* **244**: 1443–1445.

Schneider HPG (1986) The Climacteric Syndrome. In Greenblatt RD (ed.) *A Modern Approach to the Perimenopausal Years*, pp 39–55. Berlin, New York: Walter de Gruyter.

Shahrad DP & Marks R (1977) A pharmacological effect of oestrone on human epidermis. *British Journal of Dermatology* **97**: 383–386.

Sitruk-Ware R, deLignieres B, Basdevant A et al (1980) Absorption of percutaneous estradiol in postmenopausal women. *Maturitas* **2**: 202–211.

Smith P (1972) Age changes in the female urethra. *British Journal of Urology* **44**: 667–676.

Stampfer MJ, Willett WC, Colditz JA et al (1985) A prospective study of postmenopausal estrogen therapy and coronary heart disease. *New England Journal of Medicine* **313**: 1044.

Stanton SL, Oszoy A & Hilton P (1983) Voiding difficulties in the female: prevalence, clinical and urodynamic review. *Obstetrics and Gynecology* **61**: 144–147.

Stevenson JC & Whitehead MI (1982) Postmenopausal osteoporosis. *British Medical Journal* **285**: 585–588.

Strecker JB, Lauritzen CH, Nebelung J & Musch K (1980) Climacteric symptoms, estrogens and gonadotrophins in plasma and urine after application of estradiol ointment on the abdominal skin of oophorectomized women. In Mauvais-Jarvis P, Vickers CFH & Wepierre J (eds) *Percutaneous absorption of steroids*, pp 267–272.

Studd JWW & Magos A (1988) Oestrogen therapy and endometrial pathology. *The Menopause* **18**: 197–212.

Studd JWW & Parsons A (1977) Sexual dysfunction: The Climacteric. *British Journal of Sexual Medicine* **1**: 11–12.

Studd JWW & Thom M (1981) Oestrogens and endometrial cancer. In Studd JWW (ed.) *Progress in Obstetrics and Gynaecology*, pp 182–188. London: Churchill Livingstone.

Studd JWW, Collins WP, Chakravarti S, Newton JR, Oram D & Parsons A (1977) Oestradiol and Testosterone implants in the treatment of psychosexual problems in the post-menopausal woman. *British Journal of Obstetrics and Gynaecology* **84**: 314–316.

Studd JWW, Dubiel M, Kakkar W, Thom M & White PJ (1978) The effect of hormone replacement therapy on glucose tolerance, clotting factors, fibrinolysis and platelet behaviour in post-menopausal women. In Cook ID (ed.) *The Role of Oestrogen/Progestogen in the Management of the Menopause*, pp 41–59. Lancaster: MTP Press.

Studd JWW, Thom MH, Paterson NEL & Wade-Evans T (1980) The prevention and treatment of endometrial pathology in postmenopausal women receiving exogenous estrogens. In Pasetto N, Paoletti R & Ambrvs JL (ed.) *The menopause and postmenopause*, pp 127–139. Lancaster: MTP Press.

Studd JWW, Anderson HM & Montgomery JC (1986) Selection of patients—kind and duration of treatment. In Greenblatt RB (ed.) *A Modern Approach to the Postmenopausal Years*, pp 129–140. Berlin, New York: Walter de Gruyter.

Stumpf WE, Sur M & Joshi SE (1976) Estrogen target cells in the skin. **Experientia 30**: 196–199.

Sturdee DW, Wilson KA, Pipilli E & Crocker AD (1978) Physiological aspects of the menopausal hot flush. *British Medical Journal* **2**: 79–80.

Tataryn IV, Lomax P, Bajonek JG, Chesarek W, Meldrum DR & Judd HL (1980) Post-menopausal hot flushes: a disorder of thermoregulation. *Maturitas* **2**: 101–107.

Thom M, Chakravarti S, Oram DH & Studd JWW (1977) Effect of hormone replacement therapy on glucose tolerance in postmenopausal women. *British Journal of Obstetrics and Gynaecology* **84**: 776–784.

Thom M, Dubiel M, Kakkar VV, Studd JWW (1978) The effects of different regimes of oestrogen on the clotting and fibrinolytic system of the postmenopausal women. *Oestrogen Therapy. Frontiers of Hormone Research* **5**: 192–202.

Thom MH, Collins WP & Studd JWW (1981) Hormone profiles in postmenopausal women after therapy with subcutaneous implants. *British Journal of Obstetrics and Gynaecology* **88**: 426–433.

Thombom J & Oswald I (1977) Effect of oestrogen on sleep, mood and anxiety of menopausal women. *British Medical Journal* **2**: 1317–1319.

Thompson B, Hart SA & Durno D (1973) Menopausal age and symptomatology in a general practice. *Journal of Biosocial Science* **5**: 71–82.

Tiegs RD, Body JJ, Warner HW, Barta J, Riggs BL & Heath HI (1984) Calcitonin Secretion in postmenopausal osteoporosis. *New England Journal of Medicine* **312**: 1097–1100.

Tikkanen MJ, Nikkila EA, Kunsi T (1986) Lipids, hormonal status and the cardiovascular system in the menopause. In Greenblatt RB (ed.) *A Modern Approach to the Perimenopausal Years*, pp 77–86. Berlin, New York: Walter de Gruyter.

Tulandi T, Kinch RA, Guyda H, Mazella L & Lal S (1984) Effect of methyldopa on menopausal flushes, skin temperature and luteinizing hormone secretion. *American Journal of Obstetrics and Gynecology* **150**: 709–712.

Utian WH (1987) Alternative delivery systems for steroid hormones. In Zichella L, Whitehead MI & van Keep PA (ed.) *The Climacteric and Beyond*, pp 169–183. New Jersey: Parthenon Publishing Group.

Van der Meer J, Stoepman van Dalen EA & Jensen JMS (1973) Anti-thrombin III deficiency in a Dutch family. *Journal of Clinical Pathology* **26**: 532–538.

Vashinav R, Gallagher JA, Beresford NN & Russell RGG (1984) Proliferative effects of oestrogens on bone derived cells. *Calcified Tissue International* **36** (supplement 2): S59.

Versi E (1986) The bladder in the menopausal women. In Greenblatt RB (ed.) *A Modern Approach to the Perimenopausal Years*, pp 93–102. Berlin, New York: Walter de Gruyter.

Versi E & Cardozo LD (1985) Urethral vascular pulsations. *Proceedings of the International Continence Society, London*, pp 503–594.

Versi E, Cardozo LD, Brincat M, Cooper D, Montgomery JC & Studd JWW (1988) Correlation of urethral physiology and skin collagen in postmenopausal women. *British Journal of Obstetrics and Gynaecology* **95**: 147–152.

Vickers CFH (1980) Reservoir effect of human skin: pharmacological speculation. In Mautais-Jarvis P, Vickers CFH & WePierie J (eds) *Percutaneous absorption of steroids*, pp 19–20. London: Academic Press.

Voda AM (1981) Climacteric Hot Flush. *Maturitas* **3**: 73–90.

Walter S, Wolf I, Barlebo H & Jensen HK (1978) Urinary incontinence in postmenopausal women treated with oestrogens. A double blind clinical trial. *Urologia Internationalis* **33**: 136–143.

Warren MP, Brooks-Gunn J, Hamilton LH, Warren F & Hamilton J (1986) Scoliosis and fractures in young ballet dancers. *New England Journal of Medicine* **314**: 1348–1353.

Whitehead MI & Crust M (1987) Consequences and treatment of early loss of ovarian function. In Zichella C, Whitehead, M & van Keep PA (eds) *The Climacteric and Beyond*, pp 63–68. New Jersey: The Parthenon Publishing Group.

Whitehead MI & Studd JWW (1988) Selection of patients for treatment. Which therapy and for how long? *The Menopause* **10**: 116–129.

Whitehead MI, Mirandi J, Kitchin Y & Sharples MJ (1978) Systemic absorption of estrogen from Premarin vaginal cream. In Cooke ID (ed.) *The Role of Estrogen/Progestagen in the management of the menopause*, pp 63–71. Lancaster: MTP Press.

Whitehead MI, Lane G, Dyer G, Townsend PT, Collins WP & King RJB (1981) Estradiol: the predominant intranuclear estrogen in the endometrium of estrogen-treated postmenopausal women. *British Journal of Obstetrics and Gynaecology* **88**: 914–918.

Wilson PWF, Garrison RJ & Custelli WO (1985) Postmenopausal estrogen use, cigarette smoking and cardiovascular morbidity in women over 59. *New England Journal of Medicine* **313**: 1038.

5

Dermatological conditions of the vulva

C. MARJORIE RIDLEY

Most cutaneous problems of the vulva are probably best managed by the combined skills of a dermatologist and a general practitioner. It may, however, be a gynaecologist or geriatrician who initially encounters the patient, and the ensuing account is intended as a guide for this situation. More detailed considerations of all the topics will be found elsewhere (Ridley, 1988). The term dermatosis is used as a general term for any non-infective, non-neoplastic skin condition which is recognized as a dermatological entity.

GENERAL CONSIDERATIONS

Genital dermatological problems in the elderly are essentially similar to those at other times of life, but there are a few conditions and aspects of diagnosis and management which are more or less peculiar to this age group. In addition, it is important to distinguish between physical conditions in the genital area and those elsewhere. Local factors of heat, friction and occlusion modify morphology. Blisters rupture; hyperkeratosis shows as pale soggy tissue rather than as crisp and white; thickening of the epidermis is pale rather than earthy in colour; secondary infection is common. On an experimental level the skin of the labia majora is known to be more readily irritated than normal skin, to have increased transepidermal water excretion and to be more easily penetrated by hydrocortisone. These findings are relevant in considering the potential of local applications for good or ill. Furthermore, there is a transition between skin proper and mucosa as one moves from the labia majora to the labia minora and the vestibule. Such differences modify not only the morphology of any given eruption but are concerned in its pattern. Many dermatoses for example never involve mucosal surfaces.

It is particularly important to make a definitive diagnosis in a vulval lesion to avoid missing infective and neoplastic conditions. Neoplasia will clearly be suspected in the presence of a mass (and the general rule in such cases is to excise and check the histology), but may not be considered in the case of intraepithelial neoplasia (VIN) which may masquerade as a dermatosis. Both squamous and non-squamous (extramammary Paget's disease) VIN are likely to be encountered in the elderly (Figure 1a & 1b); wherever there is doubt a biopsy should be carried out. With a disposable punch biopsy a specimen can easily be obtained with local anaesthesia; multiple specimens are often indicated. Such specimens are also useful where the diagnosis of a dermatological condition is in doubt and for establishing immunofluorescence findings. This is important in the bullous disorders, where such biopsies are put into liquid nitrogen or into special transport medium.

Often several conditions co-exist and must be distinguished; a dermatosis, for example, may become infected and an allergy may develop to topical applications. Patch tests may be needed to investigate the allergy. In the elderly, underlying prolapse and incontinence may increase the complexity.

The history, especially if expanded after examination, may be valuable but some elderly patients may recount very little. The examination must be orderly and complete—not as easy as it sounds if problems of mobility and obesity exist. Other areas of the skin should be examined and the urine checked; sometimes vaginal and pelvic examination will be indicated. After the major changes of puberty and in pregnancy, the changes of the ano-

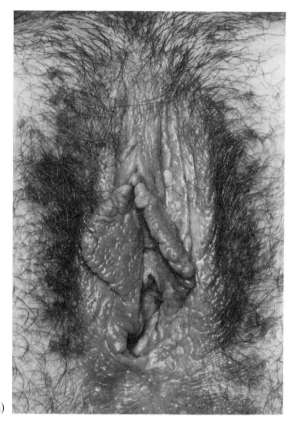

(a)

Figure 1 (a). VIN III with pigmentation. From Ridley (1988), with permission. (b) Extramammary Paget's disease: reddish/whitish lesions of anterior vulva. From Beilby and Ridley (1987), with permission.

genital area encountered in later life are more gradual and limited in their degree, but a recognition of such subtle gradations is a prerequisite of accurate diagnosis and treatment. It is important, for example, not to confuse physiological with pathological atrophy. In the elderly one must take into account the modification brought about by prolapse, caruncles and previous surgery; such minor features as episiotomy scars can cause confusion if not recognized when one is searching for some minute lesion indicated by the patient.

Although, in general, any lump should be excised or biopsied, an exception can be made for certain easily recognizable benign lesions. One example is that of sebaceous retention, perhaps with cyst formation, when single or profuse hard yellowish nodules are seen on the labia majora. Another is the small, single or multiple purplish lesion of angiomas and angiokeratomas (analogous to the Fordyce condition in the male) on the labia majora. The superficial darkish warty plaques of seborrhoeic warts on the pubic area are also usually easily recognizable and they can be left alone or curetted; if a lesion is suggestive of a mole it is probably wiser to remove it and to check the histology. Diffuse pigmentation may be puzzling; if exogenous factors (see below) are excluded, the most likely causes are post-inflammatory changes or multiple lentigines; a biopsy is usually wise if only not to miss the occasional rare case where apparently innocent pigmentation is in fact part of a VIN.

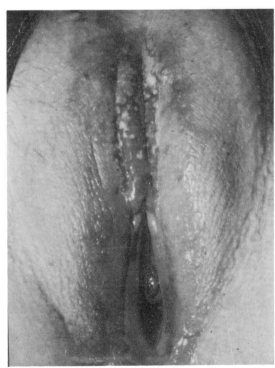

(b)

SYSTEMIC DISEASE

Glucagonoma

Almost all patients with this rare pancreatic tumour have a characteristic rash, mainly evident in the genital area. The lesions are red and blistering, showing a tendency to heal at the edge of extending affected areas. The patient is usually middle-aged or elderly and ill with extreme weight loss, glossitis and stomatitis. Diabetes is common. The serum glucagon is greatly raised. The histology shows epidermal necrolysis with a mild chronic dermal infiltrate. Management rests on treatment of the tumour and of any metastases, whereupon the rash abates.

Ulcerative colitis and Crohn's disease

Ulcerative colitis is occasionally accompanied by vegetating pustular lesions in the groins. Crohn's disease is much more often accompanied by skin lesions and these take the form of vulval swellings, sinuses, fistulae and skin tags (Figure 2). The histology may be non-specific in lymphoedematous

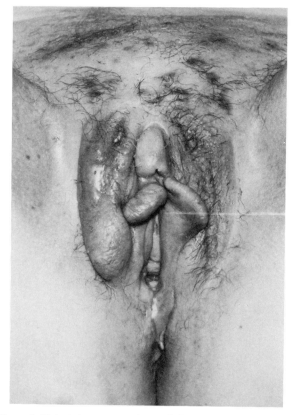

Figure 2. Vulval change secondary to inflammatory bowel disease.

cases but usually shows the typical epithelioid granulomata. Treatment of the bowel condition may help, as may limited local surgery. Topical antiseptics and corticosteroids are of some value.

Many rare systemic conditions can involve the vulva and are considered elsewhere (Ridley, 1988).

SEXUALLY TRANSMITTED DISEASES

Sexually transmitted diseases are less often encountered in this age group than in younger patients but must not be forgotten.

Warts

Genital warts may sometimes appear (or may persist), reaching large size but without evidence of malignancy; the chances of malignant transformation are probably higher in the elderly, however, and should not be overlooked; again biopsy is indicated.

Herpes simplex (and herpes zoster, not sexually transmitted)

Herpes simplex may be seen in and around the genital area either as a recurrence of a longstanding lesion, as a first attack from an infection possibly contracted long before, or as a new infection. A swab for viral culture will establish the diagnosis.

Herpes zoster is relatively common in the older age groups and if the third sacral dermatome (S_3) is affected will appear as a painful unilateral blistering rash. Infections of S_3 and sometimes those of S_2 or S_4 dermatomes may cause a neuropathic bladder disorder. Post-herpetic neuralgia is particularly liable to follow zoster in older patients. Diagnosis, if not clinically obvious, is by culture.

Management

In herpes simplex, analgesia and treatment of secondary infection is important. Acyclovir is less effective in recurrent infections (though shortening the time of shedding) than in primary ones, when it shortens the attack without affecting the rate of recurrence. The general policy now is to give intravenous acyclovir in severe infections, oral acyclovir in primary cases and the cream in mild primary attacks (Oriel, 1988).

In herpes zoster, analgesia and simple applications such as povidone iodine may be sufficient. If a more specific treatment is required, however, idoxuridine 40% in dimethylsulphoxide may be helpful in shortening inflammation, but probably not pain. The role of acyclovir has not yet been fully explored (Oriel, 1988). In both herpes simplex and herpes zoster treatment should be early and thorough in the immunosuppressed patient.

VAGINAL DISCHARGE

Any vaginal discharge may irritate vulval skin. In the elderly, a Candida vaginitis or vulvo-vaginitis is unusual except in uncontrolled diabetes, when it will present with soreness and marked swelling and erythema; discharge may be inconspicuous but if present will be thick and white. Mixed bacterial vaginosis is not uncommon. *Gardnerella vaginalis* (previously Haemophilus vaginalis or Corynebacterium vaginale) is a coccobacillus and is found in such cases, but Bacteroides and Peptococcus species are also of significance and are responsible for the typical fishy smell of the discharge. Mycoplasma hominis and Mobiluncus, a mobile rod, are also found in such cases (Oriel, 1988). Some degree of vaginal discharge may be associated with simple atrophy. Discharge may be associated with neoplasia of the lower genital tract as well as occurring as an aftermath of laser treatment or cryotherapy.

Management

In all such cases, the vulva becomes inflamed and moist and it is important to ascribe the symptoms to the correct cause and to investigate and treat them as necessary. Candida infections will respond to clotrimazole pessaries and a hydrocortisone/miconazole or clotrimazole cream; diabetes must be controlled. Mixed bacterial vaginosis is best treated with oral metronidazole (which is only partly effective against *Gardnerella* but very effective against anaerobes). Discharge in relation to hypo-oestrogenic atrophy can be remedied by local or systemic oestrogens. Sea salt baths are recommended following cryotherapy or laser surgery.

INCONTINENCE

Incontinence of urine will lead to a napkin rash type of eruption with relative sparing of folds. Secondary infection is common. Incontinence of faeces will have similar effects. If Dorbanex has been taken, the urine will stain the skin orange and the sites of faecal contamination will be rendered brown. A rash with granulomatous lumps has been described in some elderly incontinent women, possibly analogous to a certain type of napkin eruption in babies.

Management

Nursing care is all-important. Frequent turning will minimize erosion of inflamed pressure sites. To deal with the incontinence as far as possible is obviously desirable and, if the patient is in hospital, catheterization for a time is helpful. Careful washing with a mild soap and water, or with saline if the area is very inflamed, must be followed by meticulous drying. Although folds are relatively spared, it is still of value to separate them by cotton or cotton/polyester material with a view to minimizing friction of apposing surfaces.

Irritant effects of faeces and urine are often added to by secondary infection, so a hydrocortisone preparation is often best combined with an antibacterial or anticandida agent such as miconazole. In milder cases, an absorbent dusting powder may suffice or indeed the application of a bland emollient such as zinc cream. The use of a silicone-containing 'barrier' cream may be of some limited value, though probably no more so than an emollient; neither is a substitute for assiduous nursing care.

INTERTRIGO

This inflammation of folds is the consequence of heat, obsesity, sweating and friction. It is common in the ano-genital area, especially in patients who are lying in bed on rubber drawsheets. The area is red, moist and malodorous; secondary infection with bacteria and Candida is inevitable.

Management

An absorbent dusting powder, separation of folds by cotton or cotton/ polyester material, and a mild corticosteroid perhaps with an antibacterial or anticandida agent (e.g. hydrocortisone/miconazole) is usually helpful.

LABIAL ADHESIONS

It is suspected that many cases of labial adhesion go unreported. The patients present with incontinence or urinary infection because of accumu- lation of urine behind the fused tissue; 'labial adhesions' is usually a misnomer because no labial structure can be identified. A pin-hole orifice remains, usually posteriorly placed. Such cases are usually attributed to lack of oestrogens, but on no good evidence. Some may result from cicatricial pemphigoid or lichen planus (see below) but such patients tend to have other persistent symptoms and lesions. It is likely that most, if not all, are caused by lichen sclerosus (see below). The histology in these patients should be checked. Separation by surgical means is feasible but the patients must assiduously maintain the passage by emollients and dilators.

PRURITUS VULVAE

Pruritus vulvae is defined as itching without apparent cause, i.e. arising on normal skin, and it seems to be less frequently encountered now. The rubbing or scratching which supervenes leads to a marked thickening of the affected areas and is apparent especially in the labia majora. The skin becomes a pale earthy colour and the folds soggy and white. The changes are self perpetuating and are referred to as lichen simplex or lichenification (the latter term is also used for thickening which supervenes on any itching skin condition, e.g. lichenified eczema); they may occur elsewhere on the body but the genital area appears particularly susceptible to this process. The histology shows marked acanthosis with broadened papillary processes and a chronic dermal inflammatory infiltrate.

Management

Management demands resolution of the changes not only for the relief of symptoms but in order to establish whether or not there is some underlying dermatological lesion which has itched (thus removing the case from the true pruritus vulvae category); such underlying causes are commonly eczema and lichen sclerosus et atrophicus. The main approach therapeutically is to use topical corticosteroids such as hydrocortisone 2.5% or an even stronger preparation for a short period, while at the same time removing irritants and sensitizers as noted below. A mild sedative at night e.g. hydroxyzine may help. The itch/rub cycle will tend to be repeated unless the precipitating factor (anxiety, or perhaps something banal such as friction and sweating), can be discovered and dealt with. Where this is impossible the patient can use the corticosteroid to check recurrence. Very difficult and chronic cases have been treated by alcohol injections but such measures are unlikely to be necessary given current alternative modalities of treatment. Surgery is not indicated.

VULVAL DISCOMFORT

Burning and soreness without obvious objective basis is now a common complaint in young and even middle-aged women where it usually accompanies a vestibulitis of minimal physical signs and of uncertain aetiology. This picture is unusual in the elderly. Older patients may, however, complain of severe pain at the vulva, in the vagina, in the perineal or in the anal area. Such pain is usually worse on sitting, better when walking or lying flat. If local and neurological factors can be excluded (and they are rarely to be found) the most likely diagnosis is that of depression. This group seems to fall into the category sometimes described as dermatological non-disease and is perhaps similar to those with perineal neuralgia and chronic perianal pain. When they have had operations it is tempting to think in terms of 'trapped nerves' or 'scars' but this may be unrewarding and lead to further intervention and supposed cause for symptoms. Certainly attitudes common in chronic pain problems arise, whether primary or secondary in origin.

Management

Local measures such as bland emollients, topical anaesthetics (lignocaine is not likely to sensitize although others are), and a rubber ring for sitting, to ease pressure, may be of limited value, but psychiatric assessment, anti-depressants or help from a pain clinic are usually indicated. Further aspects are discussed by Bradley and Ridley (1988).

ECZEMA (DERMATITIS)

So-called constitutional eczemas, e.g. atopic and seborrhoeic dermatitis, rarely affect the vulva. Much more important is eczema caused by the irritant or allergic effects of applied substances.

Irritants include sprays and disinfectants. Allergy readily develops to many topical applications especially local anaesthetics (except lignocaine), local antihistamines and some antibiotics; other causes include scents. The skin becomes swollen and inflamed (Figure 3). Histology shows para-keratosis, epidermal spongiosis and a chronic inflammation in the dermis. Secondary infection is common. If the cause persists, marked thickening (lichenification) develops).

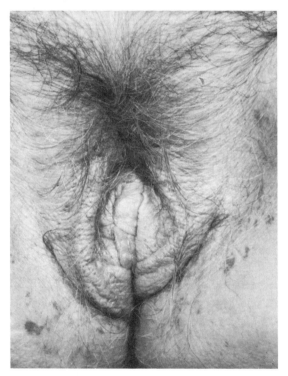

Figure 3. Eczema with thickening and secondary infection. From Beilby and Ridley (1987), with permission.

Management

All likely causes should be removed. Saline or potassium permanganate 1:10000 soaks (using a bowl or bidet) can be followed by a mild topical corticosteroid as a cream. A hair dryer or fan playing upon the area with the patient at rest in bed is helpful. For secondary infection the addition of topical miconazole or clotrimazole is useful to combat Candida and bacteria, e.g. a miconazole/hydrocortisone combination. When the condition has resolved it is important that a dermatologist should carry out patch tests if an allergy is suspected. Resolution also offers an opportunity to see if there is an underlying condition, demanding its own assessment and management, upon which an irritant or allergic dermatitis has been superimposed.

PSORIASIS

Although psoriasis typically affects extensor surfaces it may appear in flexures. Psoriasis is common, and is frequently encountered in the ano-genital area. There may or may not be lesions elsewhere and a personal or family history of the condition. The diagnosis must be made on the morphology of the lesions. Silvery scaling will often be seen in lesions of the pubic area and on the labia majora but will be absent in lesions in the genito-crural folds and perianal area; mucosal aspects are not involved. The smooth erythema and sharp outline are the important features in diagnosis. The histology shows parakeratosis, acanthosis and an absent granular layer with dermal inflammatory changes; small collections of neutrophils, the abscesses of Munro, are often seen within the epidermis. The lesions tend to be chronic and often lead to considerable anxiety and depression.

Management

A strong steroid preparation has a dramatic effect; 2.5% and, later, even 1% hydrocortisone will usually suffice for maintenance, keeping lesions to a tolerable minimum. Long-term use of stronger corticosteroid preparations may lead to stretch marks. Tar and dithranol, useful in psoriasis elsewhere, must not be used.

BEHÇET'S SYNDROME AND OTHER ULCERATIVE CONDITIONS

Behçet's syndrome may be accompanied by vulval ulcers and other systems will be involved, the full picture developing over a long period. The diagnosis is a difficult one to establish. Sporadic ulceration of other types may occur. Categorization of these ulcers is not satisfactory and histology is non-specific. They are rare in the elderly.

FIXED DRUG ERUPTION

A fixed drug eruption, though rarer in the genital area in women than in men, may affect the vulva. Likely causes are tetracycline, sulphonamides and phenolphthalein. A dull reddish fixed plaque erupts from time to time and a blister forms, subsiding to leave an area of pigmentation.

BULLOUS DISEASE

Some of the conditions characterized by bullae (i.e. blistering) have a predeliction for the vulva. Of the acute lesions, this applies to the Stevens Johnson syndrome and to some extent to toxic epidermal necrolysis; with chronic lesions, this occurs in pemphigus, cicatricial pemphigoid and benign familial chronic pemphigus.

Stevens Johnson syndrome

This variant of erythema multiforme, categorized by its mucosal involvement, is usually the result of a herpetic infection or of a reaction to a drug, most often a sulphonamide or a butazone (though use of the latter is, largely for this reason, now much curtailed). Typical iris lesions, often acral, may or may not be present; ocular and oral ulceration usually accompany genital ulceration. The subepidermal bulla is accompanied by basal cell necrosis and dermal inflammatory changes. The patient is often ill and, in the frail elderly, life is endangered. Removal of any suspected cause and skilled nursing are essential. Systemic steroids are probably contraindicated because of their side-effects and encouragement of infection.

Toxic epidermal necrolysis (TEN) and staphylococcal scalded skin syndrome (SSS)

These conditions are now separated on aetiological and histopathological grounds. TEN is commoner in adults and may be idiopathic or drug induced; SSS occurs (rarely) in this age group and especially in the immunosuppressed. Management differs between the two conditions so histology on frozen section is sometimes indicated as an emergency measure. The patient is ill, with painful necrosis of much of the body surface. The onset is often heralded by painful lesions of the perioral and perigenital area. In SSS there is a superficial split in the epidermis. In TEN there is subepidermal bulla followed by destruction of the whole epidermis. Systemic steroids are not indicated in either form. In SSS antibiotics are necessary. In both conditions, nursing care as for burns is essential.

Benign familial chronic pemphigus

This rare, genetically-determined dermatosis affects flexures. Although it often appears in the genitocrural area and outer aspects of the labia majora, it does not encroach on non-keratinized skin. The surface appears moist, fissured and reddened; frank bullae are rarely seen (Figure 4). The appearance may easily be mistaken for a banal inflamed dermatitis. Lack of resolution with simple remedies may arouse suspicion and biopsy is diagnostic; there is striking acantholysis said to resemble a dilapidated brick wall. Lesions tend to be triggered off by local infection whether bacterial, herpetic or from Candida. Management includes treatment of such factors and use of topical corticosteroids; sometimes oral antibiotics, steroids or dapsone are indicated.

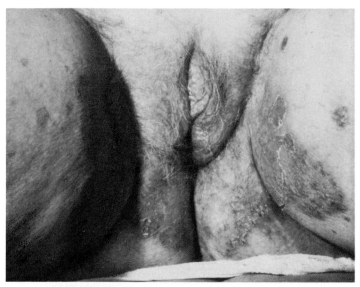

Figure 4. Benign familial chronic pemphigus: moist diffuse scaly erythema. From Beilby and Ridley (1987), with permission.

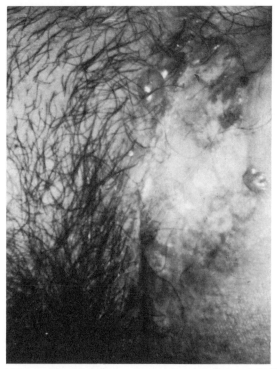

Figure 5. Cicatricial pemphigoid: bullae, scarring. From Beilby and Ridley (1987), with permission.

Cicatricial pemphigoid

Bullous pemphigoid, while relatively common in the elderly, does not often involve the vulva. Cicatricial pemphigoid however, though rarer, can affect not only cutaneous but mucosal aspects of the vulva as it does the mucosal surfaces of the eyes and mouth (Figure 5). If the tense bullae are seen, the diagnosis is relatively easy though it should always be confirmed by biopsy and immunofluorescence; when only scarring is visible it is easily confused with lichen sclerosus. The scarring may cause difficulty in micturition. Histology shows a subepidermal bulla with fibrosis, and direct immuno-fluorescence IgG along the basement membrane zone; indirect immuno-fluorescence is not always positive, but, if it is, circulating antibodies to the basement membrane zone are found. Treatment is with topical and oral steroids and often immunosuppressives, e.g. azathioprine.

Pemphigus

Pemphigus is rare and tends to begin in middle life but it is very chronic and it may also begin in the elderly. The vulval skin and mucosa are often involved and it may affect the vagina as well as skin and mucosae elsewhere. Painful flaccid bullae and eroded areas are seen (Figure 6). Histology shows an

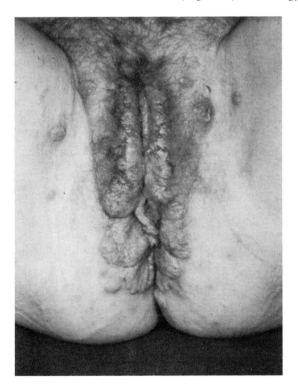

Figure 6. Pemphigus: vegetating bullous masses. From Ridley (1975), with permission.

intraepidermal vesicle with acantholysis, direct immunofluorescence IgG between the epidermal cells and indirect immunofluorescence antibodies to the inter-epidermal substance. Treatment is with high doses of steroids and immunosuppressives. Problems with side-effects are common.

With all these chronic bullous disorders management is complex and best conducted by a dermatologist.

LICHEN PLANUS

Lichen planus, a condition of uncertain aetiology but probably with an autoimmune link, usually appears on keratinized skin and in the mouth. On the skin the flat topped shiny purplish papules are easily recognized and in the mouth the milky white reticulation is characteristic. Vulval lesions are probably commoner than is thought and according to their site resemble those on the skin elsewhere or in the mouth. The histology is very specific: hyperkeratosis and acanthosis; a prominent granular layer; rather saw-toothed rete pegs; a dense band of lymphocytes in the dermis coming up to the dermo-epidermal junction, where there is often liquefaction degeneration and colloid bodies.

Management

Topical corticosteroids help the itching and lesions usually die out in a few months. Longstanding vulval lichen planus may be one of the causes of vulval atrophy and squamous carcinoma has been described in such cases.

EROSIVE LICHEN PLANUS

Although there is no hard and fast distinction between the clinical variants and 'ordinary' lichen planus may lead to mucosal lesions and to atrophy, erosive lichen planus does merit separate attention.

Early reports of lichen planus in the vagina were insubstantial, but in the last few years it has become clear that erosive lichen planus often affects vulval and vaginal mucosa, often together with erosive gingivitis, with or without 'ordinary' skin and oral lesions. The lesions at the vulva are chronic and may be premalignant (carcinoma is well recognized as a rare complication of erosive oral lesions). The areas are often extensive and are almost always extremely painful (Figure 7). Histology is difficult to obtain and often non-specific, so establishing the diagnosis may take some time and will rest on the presence and histology of lesions elsewhere. The main point of interest for the gynaecologist is that the vaginal signs and symptoms may predominate and the rest of the picture may escape attention. The vaginal mucosa tends to be friable and haemorrhagic; pain and bleeding on intercourse are common complaints. Synechiae form and the walls fuse together. Operation will be followed by prompt recurrence. Examination and the taking of cervical smears may be extremely difficult or impossible.

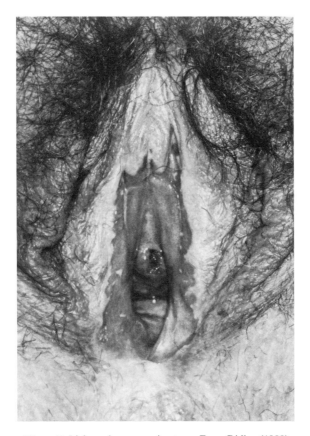

Figure 7. Lichen planus: erosive type. From Ridley (1988).

Management

Local application of topical corticosteroids in some form can be attempted, e.g. hydrocortisone (Colifoam). Oral steroids are sometimes helpful. Other agents used empirically, e.g. dapsone, griseofulvin and etretinate are, at best, of doubtful value. Surgical excision with or without grafting can be helpful in eroded lesions of the mouth, hands and feet and has been contemplated at the vulva and vagina in desperate cases.

LICHEN SCLEROSUS ET ATROPHICUS (LSA)

A large proportion of elderly women with a vulval complaint will be found to have LSA, a condition of great interest from many points of view—its aetiology, clinical manifestations, relationship to malignancy and central role in old controversies on terminology are all important. The main point to bear in mind is the existence of LSA as an entity, so that it is viewed, shorn of all anxieties over confusing nomenclature, just as one would regard, for example, eczema or psoriasis. Some of the historical discussions are summarized elsewhere (Ridley, 1988).

The aetiology is essentially unknown; a link with autoimmune disease is well substantiated (Meyrick Thomas et al, 1988); defects in elastin metabolism and local hormonal abnormalities have been postulated but the evidence is not conclusive.

The lesions of LSA, which affect all areas of the body, at all ages and in both sexes, have a characteristic appearance clinically and histologically. In a series of 350 women with proven LSA (Meyrick Thomas et al, 1988), 97.5% had vulval, 53.5% vulval and anal, and 18% lesions elsewhere with or without ano-genital lesions. The lesions are ivory-white papules often with a central depression, and they may coalesce into plaques in which purplish speckling and frank purpura are common. The vulva is affected in a variety of ways; small whitish patches on any aspect of the labia minora, whiteness and purpura of the clitoris and of the prepuce, which is often fused over, or generalized whiteness, atrophy and speckling of the labia minora; the inner aspect of the labia majora is usually spared but white papules may be seen on the extensor aspects and sometimes lesions affect the genito-crural folds, the natal cleft and the mons pubis. In some patients the pallor may be intense

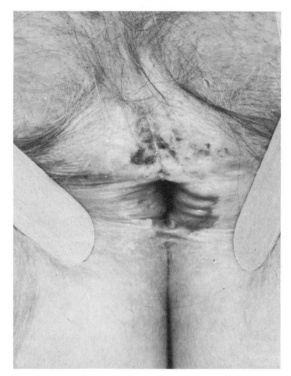

Figure 8. LSA; atrophy, loss of contours, speckling. From Beilby and Ridley (1987), with permission.

and textural changes minimal, thus making the differential diagnosis from vitiligo important. Crinkly atrophy or sclerosis may dominate and there is often a waxy yellowish colour of the severely affected labia minora (Figure 8). Where there is perianal involvement, a figure-of-eight pattern is seen. Occasionally, all traces of normal contours are obliterated and only a pin-hole meatus remains (Figure 9). This may account for many, if not all, cases described as labial adhesions in the elderly (see above).

Itching and rubbing lead to a paradoxically thickened picture and the presence of underlying LSA will be realized only when this lichenification has been resolved (Figure 10). Another manifestation is a thick hyperkeratotic honeycomb-like plaque, perhaps most often seen at the introitus in patients who have had a vulvectomy. The changes may cause introital stenosis and dyspareunia but do not extend into the vagina. Itching may be distressing, mild or totally absent. Soreness and burning may mean secondary infection, a combination with a vestibulitis or depression (see above).

The clinical picture and the histological appearance are varied, but there are several cardinal features in the latter enabling recognition (Figure 11).

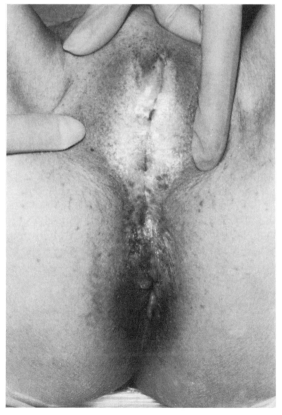

Figure 9. LSA: obliteration of contours, fusion to leave tiny orifice. From Ridley (1988), with permission.

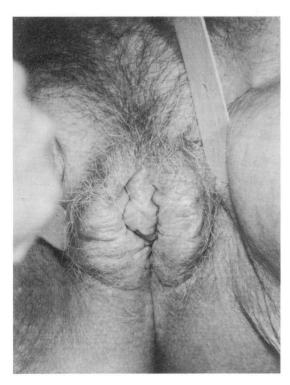

Figure 10. LSA: thickening (from rubbing) superimposed on atrophy. From Ridley (1988), with permission.

The epidermis is usually atrophic but may be hyperkeratotic in early stages and in some inflamed lesions, and acanthotic where there has been much rubbing. In such cases the rete processes tend to become elongated and forked. A subepidermal homogenous hyalinized band is typical of LSA; in it there are often extravasated red blood cells. There is a dermal band-like infiltrate of chronic inflammatory type. The histology makes clear the clinical tendency to bleeding, for the blood vessels are not supported in the normal way.

Management

Because of the link with autoimmune disease, patients should be screened for thyroid disease, diabetes and pernicious anaemia. Some patients are symptomless and need no treatment. Others have mild itching, easily controlled with bland emollients such as aqueous cream and a mild corticosteroid, e.g. hydrocortisone 1%. Stronger preparations are appropriate for short periods. Secondary infection can be dealt with using a local antibiotic or antiseptic. Patients should be reassured that the condition is not infectious or malignant and may be helped by being given some information in leaflet form.

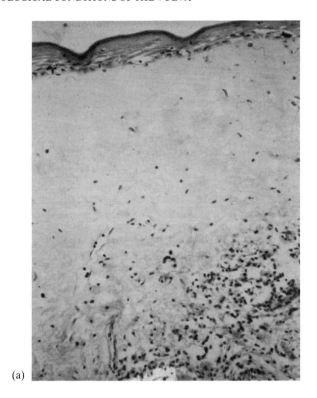

(a)

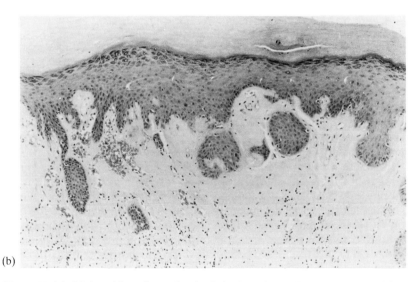

(b)

Figure 11 (a). LSA: epidermal atrophy, hyalinization; deep inflammatory band. (b) LSA: hyperkeratosis, thickened epidermis pointed rete ridges, hyalinization.

Some patients may continue to have symptoms and, especially where atrophy is predominant, local testosterone ointment (1.6% in petrolatum or some other suitable base, e.g. Unguentum Merck) may help; a course of several weeks is indicated. Testosterone ointment has found more favour in the USA than in the UK. It may act through some specifically hormonal mechanism or as a non-specific thickening agent. Large hyperkeratotic areas can usually be melted away with a strong topical corticosteroid. Persistently thickened or eroded and unhealing areas should be biopsied or excised. The laser has been used to remove troublesome areas and the recurring disease said to be more susceptible to treatment but this seems a clumsy method of management and is not recommended (Kaufman and Friedrich, 1985). Vulvectomy is followed by recurrence at the edges and should never be done in the absence of malignancy.

MALIGNANCY AND LSA

The risk of a patient with LSA developing a squamous cell carcinoma (SCC) is in the order of 5% (Meyrick Thomas et al, 1988) which appears to be significantly more than in the normal population (although many patients with LSA may never be diagnosed nor reported as such). Potentially carcinogenic radiotherapy, given in the past for pruritus, is relevant in very few.

Current views on the cause of the malignancy have swung from incriminating atrophy per se, or chronic irritation from itching (malignancy may be seen in totally symptomless LSA), to the possibility of human papillomavirus (HPV) infection. The latter, especially types 16 and 18, is clearly involved in VIN, and some VIN becomes invasive; cases are recognized where warts on LSA in the elderly become malignant (Ridley, 1986). However, most cancer in LSA appears to arise apparently de novo. Such circumstances of course do not exclude HPV as a factor and the question may not be resolved until methods are available for studying the presence and the type of HPV in malignant tissue, in surrounding tissue and, most important, in LSA without malignancy and in normal subjects. Equally, other factors may be involved, the presence of the HPV being coincidental or only part of the story. Even if the HPV turns out to be causally concerned it may well not explain all cases seen now, let alone those in the past when it seems likely that the HPV was less prevalent. Clinically, it has been accepted that inflamed, thickened LSA with fissuring and hyperkeratosis, and a histology showing what in the old ISSVD terminology was called mixed dystrophy, in the new ISSVD classification LSA and squamous hyperplasia, and in simple descriptive dermatological terms LSA and lichenification (see below) is at risk of developing into a carcinoma. As noted above, however, squamous carcinoma may arise on quite symptomless lesions. Indeed, Newton et al (1987) found that aneuploidy, usually thought to be a predictor of malignancy, was found in four out of seventeen cases of LSA; while three of the four exhibited worrying clinical and histological features, the other one (a personal case) did not. A recent paper (Evans et al, 1987) reported an interesting distinction between skin at the vulva in women with VIN and those with squamous carcinoma without any VIN; in the former group the DNA appeared abnormal only in the region of the neoplasia; in the latter it appeared unstable over a wide area, perhaps contrary to expectations when VIN is so often multifocal and SCC usually single. The practical corollary is that all cases should be kept under the supervision of an interested dermatologist or gynaecologist alert to changing appearances and aware of the need to biopsy any area which suggests neoplasia.

CLASSIFICATION

This in the past has been a confused and recriminatory area. Recent developments have remedied this; the new classification will be noted after a brief summary of past problems. Those interested in the background will find it discussed in detail elsewhere (Ridley, 1988).

Vulval conditions were first adequately described in the late nineteenth century. In retrospect many names attributed to conditions not easily categorized appear to have been LSA and lichenification (either on LSA or as the usual sequel to itching on otherwise normal skin). In 1962 Jeffcoate and Woodcock drastically simplified matters by introducing the concept of chronic epithelial dystrophy, a concept taken up by the International Society for the Study of Vulvar Disease (ISSVD) in its well-known scheme of 1976 (Table 1). Here, the stress was on histological findings. The dermato-

Table 1. Vulval dystrophies.

I. Hyperplastic dystrophy
A. Without atypia
B. With atypia
II. Lichen sclerosus
III. Mixed dystrophy (lichen sclerosus with foci of epithelial hyperplasia)
A. Without atypia
B. With atypia

Detailed histological definitions and descriptions were given of each condition noted above; atypia was classified as mild, moderate or severe, with or without dystrophy.

logists translated hyperplastic dystrophy without atypia as lichenification and mixed dystrophy as LSA with lichenification; hyperplastic dystrophy plus atypia suggests intraepithelial neoplasia.

Meanwhile, a new classification for vulval intraepithelial neoplasia (VIN) was agreed by the ISSVD and the International Society of Gynecological Pathologists (ISGYP) in 1983 and is now well accepted (Table 2). It recognizes the possible accompaniment of HPV and the importance of the general status of the patient. In 1987, discussions having continued, a new classification for non-neoplastic disorders was ratified by the ISSVD and will be accepted also by the ISGYP (Table 3). Explanatory footnotes give further details and also provide a bridge for those used to the former classification.

Table 2. Vulval intra-epithelial neoplasia (VIN).

Squamous VIN	
VIN I	Mild dysplasia
VIN II	Moderate dysplasia
VIN III	Severe dysplasia or carcinoma in situ
Non-squamous VIN	
Paget's disease	

Table 3. Non-neoplastic epithelial disorders of vulval skin and mucosa.

1. Lichen sclerosus
2. Squamous cell hyperplasia (formerly hyperplastic dystrophy)
3. Other dermatoses

The first states

'mixed epithelial disorders may occur. In such cases it is recommended that both conditions be reported. For example lichen sclerosus with associated squamous cell hyperplasis (formerly classified as mixed dystrophy) should be reported as lichen sclerosus and squamous cell hyperplasia. Squamous cell hyperplasia with associated vulval intraepithelial neoplasia (formerly hyperplastic dystrophy with atypia) should be diagnosed as vulval intraepithelial neoplasia.'

The second takes the form

'squamous cell hyperplasia is used for those instances in which the hyperplasia is not attributable to another cause. Specific lesions or dermatoses involving the vulva (e.g. psoriasis, lichen planus, lichen simplex chronicus, candida infection, condyloma acuminatum) may include squamous cell hyperplasia, but should be diagnosed specifically and excluded from this category'.

For a while, at least, agreement has been reached. A common classification will enable all concerned to compare profitably both clinical and pathological material and to standardize prospective surveys using the same terms. The 'loss' of much reported material in the past, because of lack of comparability, should not recur.

SUMMARY

Management of vulval conditions in the elderly will present no special problems if the following points are borne in mind:

1. The patient's condition will often be multifactorial; the components should be unravelled and the patient followed until the picture is clear.
2. Point 1 is particularly important because infections and neoplasia can easily go unrecognized.
3. Biopsy will often be needed.
4. Management of chronic dermatological conditions (especially where systemic treatment is indicated) is usually best carried out by the dermatologist.

5. It is vital to consider the area as one would any other as regards diagnosis of cutaneous and mucosal lesions. With this approach the vast majority of lesions can be accurately named and reasonable treatment given. To this end the naked-eye morphology, and the histopathological evidence which will sometimes be a necessary supplement, must be accurately described and understood.
6. The study of vulval conditions is interdisciplinary.
7. Much old and contentious terminology is now obsolete. The new classification is simple and should be universally applied by gynaecologists, dermatologists and pathologists so that other involved clinicians are helped rather than confused.

REFERENCES

Beilby JOW & Ridley CM (1987) The pathology of the vulva. In Fox H (ed.) *Haines and Taylor's Gynaecological and Obstetrical Pathology*. Edinburgh: Churchill Livingstone.

Bradley JJ & Ridley CM (1988) Historical and psychological considerations: Subjective and traumatic conditions of the vulva. In Ridley CM (ed.) *The Vulva*. London: Churchill Livingstone.

Evans AS, Monaghan JM & Anderson MC (1987) A nuclear deoxyribonucleic acid analysis of normal and abnormal vulvar epithelium. *Obstetrics and Gynecology* **69**: 790–793.

Kaufman RH & Friedrich EG (1985) The carbon dioxide laser in the treatment of vulvar disease. *Clinical Obstetrics and Gynecology* **28**: 220–229.

Meyrick Thomas RH, Ridley CM, McGibbon DH & Black MM (1988) Lichen Sclerosus and autoimmunity—a study of 350 women. *British Journal of Dermatology* **118**: 41–46.

Newton JA, Camplejohn RS & McGibbon DH (1987) A flow cytometric study of the significance of DNA aneuploidy in cutaneous lesions. *British Journal of Dermatology* **117**: 169–174.

Oriel JD (1988) In Ridley CM (ed.) *The Vulva*, p 78. London: Churchill Livingstone.

Ridley CM (1975) *The Vulva. Major Problems in Dermatology 5*. London: W. B. Saunders.

Ridley CM (1986) Genital warts with malignant transformation and in association with lichen sclerosus et atrophicus (LSA) in elderly women: 2 cases. *Journal of Reproductive Medicine* **31**: 984–985.

Ridley CM (1988) General dermatological conditions and dermatoses of the vulva. In Ridley CM (ed). *The Vulva*, p 138. London: Churchill Livingstone.

6

Urinary incontinence

JAMES MALONE-LEE

The last decade has seen a marked improvement in our understanding of the pathophysiology of urinary incontinence in the elderly. We are now able to manage this problem much more effectively.

The changes responsible for the development of urinary incontinence in the elderly are complex. There is no doubt that some aspects of ageing of the lower urinary tract are yet to be fully understood. Much of the work conducted to date involves cross-sectional sampling of populations with comparison between age groups (Carlile et al, 1987). If a difference exists between the elderly and the young sampled, however, it is not necessarily valid to attribute this to the ageing process: differences may have been induced by intercurrent illnesses or environmental influences. To obtain data on the changes genuinely induced by the ageing process requires longitudinal studies following people as they grow old—logistically this type of work is extraordinarily difficult to perform. In consequence the data that we do have from longitudinal studies comes from animal experiments, chiefly in mice (Phillips and Davies, 1980). It is difficult to feel confident about extrapolating the conclusions from these experiments to humans. Nevertheless we find that the elderly do exhibit different patterns of disease from those of the young. All that we can say about these observations is that they appear to be associated with old age while not necessarily being caused by natural ageing.

The detrusor muscle is a remarkably organized structure which is capable of a number of intricate functions. During filling of the bladder the detrusor relaxes as the bladder wall distends so that a virtually constant minimal pressure is maintained. The sensation of bladder fullness is transmitted to the consciousness when appropriate and not before. Contraction of the detrusor is voluntarily induced and results in a rise in bladder pressure, a closure of the ureteric orifices and opening of the bladder neck. The voiding detrusor contraction is closely coordinated with urethral sphincter relaxation and the whole process of voiding is carefully sustained until complete bladder emptying. A breakdown in one or more of these functions may lead to urinary incontinence.

Much of the normal behaviour of the bladder and urethra is dependent on complex neurological controls. Because the nervous system is particularly susceptible to age-related degenerative changes, it should be no surprise to learn that the urinary incontinence of late life has much to do with the neurology of the lower urinary tract.

ANATOMY

The external urethral sphincter is the site of maximum urethral resistance (Griffiths, 1980). As well as a resting tone it contracts reflexly in response to abdominal straining. The circularly arranged muscle fibres are striated and slow twitch in character. The positive pressure generated in the urethra during abdominal straining originates partly from direct transmission to the intra-abdominal urethra and partly from reflex sphincter contractions. The external sphincter is separate from the striated muscle of the pelvic sling which passes laterally to the urethra before inserting into the inferior pubic rami. The sling supports the bladder and proximal urethra posteriorly. If the support provided by the pelvic sling fails, urethral incompetence is likely to develop. As the bladder neck drops, the ability to transmit abdominal pressure rises to the proximal urethra becomes compromised; in addition, reflex contraction of the sphincter muscle becomes less efficient.

Continence is usually maintained at the bladder neck as a result of its position in the abdominal cavity and because of passive closure promoted by the smooth muscle and elastic tissue. The external sphincter supports this continence mechanism but will play a more significant role if the bladder neck becomes incompetent. Apart from the influence of the sphincter and the position of the urethra, continence is also promoted by the urethral elastic tissue, the pressure exerted by intramural arterio-venous sinuses, the smooth muscle of the urethral walls, and the surface tension of the mucous (Hald, 1984).

PHARMACOLOGICAL ANATOMY

Most of the detrusor fibres carry muscarinic cholinergic receptors which are innervated by parasympathetic efferents originating in the intermediolateral columns of sacral segments S_2, S_3 and S_4. Stimulation of these neurones results in a contraction. There are a number of other receptors within the detrusor but their clinical significance is limited (Malone-Lee, 1983).

The bladder neck and internal sphincter are supplied with a number of excitatory $\alpha 1$ receptors, some excitatory cholinergic receptors and a few inhibitory $\beta 2$ receptors. The smooth muscle of the urethra has a similar receptor distribution (Gosling et al, 1981). Cholinergic and α-adrenergic stimulation cause a rise in pressure at the membranous urethra.

The female urethra has oestrogen receptors throughout its length with maximum concentration in the distal two thirds (Wilson et al, 1981). Progesterone receptors have not been detected although there is a sensitivity of the urethra to progesterone (Caine and Raz, 1973).

NEUROPHYSIOLOGY

Afferent pathway function

The most important receptors in the bladder are tension receptors. The afferents which pass to the lumbar segments of the cord are concentrated in the muscle coats and submucosa of the bladder neck and urethra. Afferents going to the sacral cord are distributed throughout the bladder. The receptors respond, with varying thresholds, to tension produced by distension or contraction (Fletcher and Bradley, 1978).

The sacral afferent nerves are stimulated at low bladder volumes. They activate a sacral reflex which inhibits detrusor excitation thereby filling without a related rise in pressure (Figure 1). This reflex fails in the presence

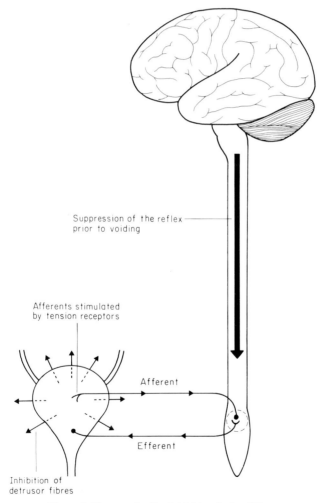

Suppression of the reflex prior to voiding

Afferents stimulated by tension receptors

Afferent

Efferent

Inhibition of detrusor fibres

Figure 1. The sacral reflex inhibiting during filling.

of a sensory neuropathy and the bladder loses compliance. The lumbar afferents respond to the extremes of distension. All tension afferents ascending to the brain do so in the lateral dorsal columns.

Some sacral afferents are involved in a different reflex arc. The sensory neurones synapse with motor efferents either at sacral level or, more importantly, after traversing the spinal cord to the pontine reticular formation. This reflex, when activated, initiates micturition and is essential for voiding. It is usually suppressed by the influence of neurones from higher cerebral centres (Figure 2).

The sensations of bladder fullness, touch and pain are conveyed from receptors in the submucosa via sacral and lumbar afferents up into the spinothalamic tracts with one third crossing to the opposite side.

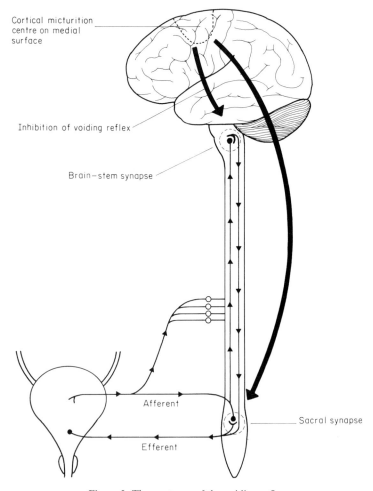

Cortical micturition
centre on medial
surface

Inhibition of voiding reflex

Brain–stem synapse

Afferent

Efferent

Sacral synapse

Figure 2. The anatomy of the voiding reflex.

Central nervous system control

An excellent review of the functional neuroanatomy of the lower urinary tract has been published by Fletcher and Bradley (1978), where more details on this subject can be obtained.

The highest centre involved in the control of micturition is located on the supero-medial aspect of both frontal lobes adjacent to the genu of the corpus callosum. This area of the hemisphere is occasionally referred to as the frontal lobe centre for micturition. It receives input from the brain-stem nuclei and the ascending tracts. Impulses pass from the frontal lobe centre to other parts of the cortex, cross the corpus callosum, or descend in the internal capsule to the brain-stem nuclei and reticulo-spinal tracts. If the cortical micturition centre is stimulated experimentally the detrusor becomes activated but the brain-stem nuclei associated with bladder control become inhibited.

The thalamus relays sensory signals from bladder, urethral and pelvic receptors, to the cortical micturition centres. Other impulses are transmitted to brain centres which are responsible for promoting a modification in behaviour in response to bladder filling.

Motor efferents from the cortical centres synapse in the basal ganglia which send communications to the brain-stem motor nuclei. Electrical stimulation of the basal ganglia in experimental animals leads to suppression of the detrusor. Ablation of the basal ganglia results in bladder hyper-reflexia.

The main brain-stem motor nuclei governing detrusor activity are situated in the pontine reticular formation. Stimulation of these nuclei results in precipitant detrusor activity whereas ablation leads to detrusor inactivity. The descending pathways from the brain-stem motor nuclei become organized into three important tracts. Nerves originating in the pons, medulla oblongata and mid-brain pass in the lateral spino-reticular tract to the motor nuclei for the sacral cord. They promote a sustained contraction of the detrusor with inhibition of the sphincters. Another group of fibres pass from the pons in the medial reticulospinal tract and inhibit the external sphincter. The third group of neurones arise in the medulla oblongata and travel in the anterior reticulospinal tract and inhibit the detrusor and stimulate the sphincters.

ASSESSING LOWER URINARY TRACT FUNCTION

Although taking the clinical history of and examining the elderly does not differ greatly from practices adopted for the young, there are some aspects which demand more attention. Some of the most frequently identified factors which may aggravate or precipitate incontinence include: immobility, impaired dexterity, poor eyesight, mental impairment and communication problems. Chronic constipation is almost invariable in the immobile and aggravates detrusor instability and any of the voiding problems. Diuretics and sedatives are notorious precipitants of incontinence. The patient's environment may need careful checking. What is the distance to the lavatory? Are there any obstacles in the way? Is the lavatory easy to identify? Is it well lit? Is it warm? Are the patient's bed and chairs suitable? The attitude of the caring staff to the incontinence is also relevant, as are the type of practices being adopted by them.

Common complications of incontinence include skin excoriation and maceration, and the use of fluid restriction in one way or another. Problems associated with odour must be identified and it is important to enquire about laundry facilities and the financial consequences of the incontinence. The ability of the relatives or carers to manage the patient's incontinence is an important part of the social assessment as incontinence is often invoked as the precipitant of a crisis within the support system. Incontinence often causes some form of social isolation and problems with self-respect. The associated depression may compromise the ability to recover.

The assessment has to involve private interviews with the patient alone and together with carers. Liaison with physiotherapists, occupational therapists and social workers is recommended as their help is often invaluable. It may be helpful to observe the patient's toileting skills in the home environment. The clinical assessment has to include a measurement of the post-micturition residual urine volume. It is also worth performing an abdominal X-ray as this is a most accurate way of screening for colonic faecal loading.

The application of the principles described above will lead to an accurate diagnosis of the cause of incontinence in an overwhelming majority of cases (Hilton and Stanton, 1981; Castleden et al, 1981a). There is no real need to submit all patients to a urodynamic investigation. In my department we use urodynamics only in the following circumstances:

1. Whenever surgery is being considered.
2. In the presence of a voiding problem.
3. When first-line treatment has failed.

The basic urodynamic investigation using pressure-flow cystometry or video cystometry has been described in a number of texts (e.g. Turner-Warwick and Whiteside, 1979; Griffiths, 1980). The investigation, though apparently simple, requires some experience if it is to be performed properly. The interpretation of the results is a skilled process and should not be taken lightly. There is no doubt that properly performed and interpreted urodynamic investigations can greatly enhance effective management.

MECHANISMS OF URINARY INCONTINENCE

With increasing age there is a reduction in bladder capacity. The voiding flow rate also reduces and there is a tendency to less complete emptying. Changes in the ability to generate bladder pressure rises vary among individuals; a reduction in bladder power is not a universal experience of the old (Resnick et al, 1985).

Urinary tract infection

A significant bacteriuria is defined by Kass and Brumfitt (1978) as at least 10^5 organisms per ml in three successive fresh, clean-catch, mid-stream specimens of urine. This provides a 95% confidence level that there is a genuine infection. One specimen fulfilling the criteria gives an 80% confidence level. The presence of more than 10 white blood cells per ml of urine indicates an inflammatory process.

Asymptomatic bacteriuria is a common finding. About 3% of women aged 25 have bacteriuria. The incidence increases by 1–2% for each decade of age reaching 7% at 65 and 9% at 85 in ambulant women. Asymptomatic bacteriuria has an incidence of 2–3% in men aged 60 to 70 and 21–30% in those over the age of 80. Any abnormality of the urinary tract will greatly increase the incidence of bacteriuria (Dontas, 1984). A urine specimen taken from a patient with a genuine infection in an average clinic will yield a significant culture about 50% of the time. If the urine specimen is clear a positive culture is even less likely. Negative cultures do not rule out genuine infection.

An acute urinary tract infection causing frequency and dysuria may well precipitate urge incontinence that resolves with treatment of the infection. The treatment of significant bacteriuria in the absence of these symptoms is not likely to improve incontinence and need only be pursued if other indications exist.

Detrusor instability

Detrusor instability or unstable bladder is the second most common cause of incontinence in all women. Its incidence increases with age. Eighty four per cent of the elderly attending my unit with urinary incontinence have been found to have unstable bladders.

Instability can be caused by damage or failure of the pathways functioning to inhibit the voiding reflex and by local disease of the bladder. Detrusor instability may be precipitated by virtually any neurological disease or trauma above the sacral cord. 'Idiopathic detrusor instability' describes the condition in the absence of a clear cause, a comparative rarity among the elderly.

The symptoms of detrusor instability comprise frequency, nocturia, urgency, urge incontinence and nocturnal enuresis. The detrusor is inadequately suppressed and tends to contract inappropriately resulting in expression of part of the bladder contents.

The bladder retraining regime is the simplest way of treating the unstable bladder and it is very effective. The patient maintains a simple bladder diary chart recording, with a tick, each micturition or episode of incontinence and works hard at increasing the intervals between micturitions. It is not logical to use fixed time intervals as normal micturition patterns are irregular. I advise patients to delay voiding for as long as possible whenever a sense of urgency develops. Once a minimum interval of four hours can be achieved the symptoms related to instability usually resolve. Retraining at night disrupts sleep and is not necessary.

The use of certain drugs can be extremely helpful as an adjuvant to the retraining regime. Though many preparations have been advocated there are, in fact, few that have been shown to be genuinely effective. The tricyclic antidepressant imipramine has anticholinergic, α-agonistic, antihistaminic and anti-5-HT properties. It has been shown to be effective for detrusor instability in a number of clinical trials. Most patients respond to a single daily dose of 10 to 20 mg at night. Some people with troublesome daytime symptoms require a morning dose as well. The dose-response varies among individuals and some people require high doses of 100 mg or more, but this is rare. Side-effects can be attributed to the anticholinergic properties—a dry mouth and constipation being common problems (Castleden et al, 1981b).

Oxybutinin is a tertiary amine with powerful anticholinergic and papaverine-like properties (Moisey et al, 1980). This drug is well absorbed and highly effective at suppressing unstable detrusor activity but its use is limited by marked anticholinergic side-effects which make it difficult to tolerate. It is given in a dose ranging from 2.5 mg o.d. to 5 mg t.d.s. Because of the side-effects the use of this drug for the elderly has its limitations but nevertheless is useful in problematic circumstances.

Terodiline is a calcium ion antagonist with anticholinergic, smooth muscle relaxant and local anaesthetic properties (Klarskov et al, 1986). It is rapidly absorbed from the gastrointestinal tract but has a very long half-life of up to 60 hours, and up to 130 hours in the frail elderly. This means that steady-state levels are not reached for at least 14 days. It seems to be well tolerated with side-effects which are not particularly severe. These involve a dry mouth, constipation and a fall in postural blood pressure.

Propantheline bromide, emepronium bromide, flavoxate hydrochloride, and non-steroidal anti-inflammatories have all been advocated for the unstable bladder but responses have not proved very impressive. The first two are quaternary ammonium compounds which do not readily pass biological membranes, making their absorption variable and often necessitating high doses.

Voiding problems

An underactive bladder may develop as a result of lesions of the sacral nerves and peripheral neuropathies. The symptoms feature: difficulties in initiating micturition, a poor urinary stream, an intermittent stream, incomplete emptying, stress incontinence and persistent dribbling incontinence. Recurrent urinary infection is another feature. Nowadays, the use of intermittent catheterization to manage an underactive bladder is a favoured approach (Lapides, 1976). It will be described later.

I have described the descending spinal pathway which bears neurones that function to sustain the micturition process once it has been initiated. If these nerves fail, voiding is incomplete and a persistent residual urine will result. This problem is usually accompanied by detrusor instability and the incontinence that results will not resolve until the voiding problem has been corrected. In addition it may only become evident because of exacerbation of symptoms or retention developing after the introduction of anticholinergic medication for an instability. An unsustained detrusor contraction is a feature of many diseases of the central nervous system, most notably multiple sclerosis, cerebrovascular disease, Alzheimer's disease and spinal injury. The treatment is intermittent catheterization. Many patients re-establish normal voiding after a short period.

A failure of coordination between detrusor and sphincter mechanisms can lead to voiding being compromised by inappropriate sphincter contractions. This is called detrusor–sphincter dyssynergia. It is more commonly seen in younger patients and rarely plays an important role in the voiding problems of the elderly.

Urethral sphincter incompetence

The symptom of stress incontinence involves urinary leakage in association with coughing, laughing, running and other similar activities. It is most commonly associated with urethral incompetence when it is referred to as genuine stress incontinence. Failure of the urethral sphincter mechanisms is frequently related to childbirth but nevertheless occurs in 5–15% of nulliparous women. Lower-motor-neurone lesions of the sacral efferents to the urethra may cause stress incontinence in the elderly, usually in association with an underactive bladder. A cough may precipitate an unstable detrusor contraction. In consequence a detrusor instability can mimic the symptoms of urethral incompetence.

Mild symptoms of genuine stress incontinence associated with minor anatomical defects will respond to pelvic floor exercises. Where this approach does not succeed then surgery should be adopted after urodynamic assessment. The preferred operation is a colposuspension but a sling procedure may also be used (Stanton, 1984). Age should not preclude women from being offered such operations.

Although oestrogenization is important for normal urethral function, topical or systemic replacement therapy has not been proven as definitely effective in treating stress incontinence.

MANAGEMENT TECHNIQUES

Pelvic floor exercises

Pelvic floor exercises are only likely to benefit women with mild stress incontinence associated with minimal descent of the bladder neck. They are also helpful to those women who present with a low pressure detrusor instability in the presence of a low urethral resistance. The grosser forms of urethral sphincter incompetence require surgical solutions.

I teach the patients to identify accurately an effective contraction of the periurethral striated muscle. I insert a finger into the vagina and identify the urethra. The patient is then encouraged to contract the periurethral muscles by mimicking the actions used to terminate micturition in mid-stream. An effective contraction can be detected by the instructor's palpating finger.

Once this has been achieved the patient is asked to remember the actions and feelings associated with the contraction. She is advised to perform this contraction, in repetitions of five, regularly throughout the day every time she turns on a tap. The use of a tap is usually associated with bladder awareness in those with an incontinence problem. If the exercises are performed adequately an ache is experienced in the perineum during the first two weeks. A response in the symptoms is usually noted over the ensuing two to three months.

Intermittent catheterization

Intermittent catheterization is an important method of managing the voiding problems described earlier in this chapter. The clean, non-sterile technique described by Lapides (1976) is the approach now widely adopted. It is not difficult to use the technique with the elderly. I teach the patient or consort to pass a CH12 plastic Jacques catheter into the bladder during a single out-patient attendance. The technique is then practised at home daily for two weeks while using antibiotic cover and 1% lignocaine jelly as lubricant. After two weeks catheterizations can usually be achieved without difficulty and a regime best suited to the individual is then developed. A bland lubricant jelly is used and catheters are passed with a frequency that keeps the patient continent, free from infection and the residual urine below 500 ml. The catheter is rinsed after each catheterization and stored in a clean polythene container to be reused and then changed at weekly intervals. Regular review of this type of management is essential and the patient must have good access to nursing and medical help if problems, though rare, should occur. If a patient is unable to perform the procedure and a consort is not available, then a district nurse may need to be involved.

Incontinence aids

A hand-held female urinal is of proven use to women with mobility problems and difficulty in getting out of bed to pass urine (Figure 3). It can be easily emptied into a bucket or commode placed by the bed.

Women who are mobile and independent are best served with a small pad which is easily stored and disposed of. The Kanga Lady systems and the Kylie pants are good examples of popular and successful products (Figures 4 and 5).

Immobile and less independent patients usually require a larger pad, such as the Molnlycke Tenaform range (Figure 6). Special front-opening pants like the Brevet Sanitas range may prove more appropriate for wheelchair bound patients who change their own pads.

The disposable bed-pad is a time-honoured method of managing incontinence at night. Usually several are required to provide adequate protection and there are problems with leakage and patient discomfort. Nowadays there are better alternatives to use during the night. There are a number of reusable bed covers which are proving to be effective, comfortable and cost-effective.

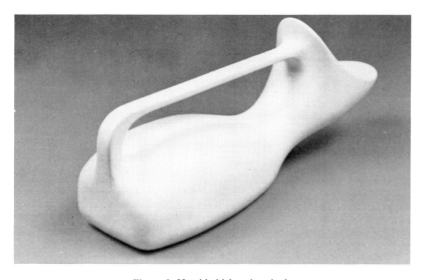

Figure 3. Hand held female urinal.

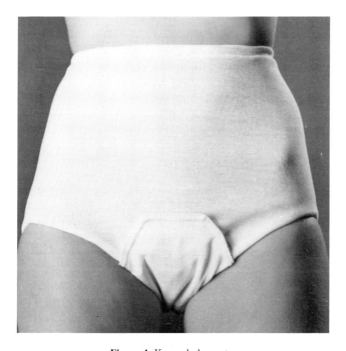

Figure 4. Kanga lady pants.

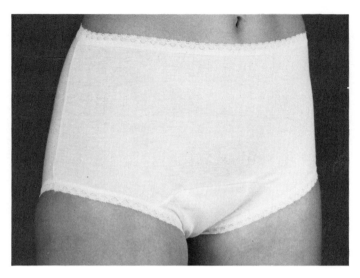

Figure 5. Kylie pants.

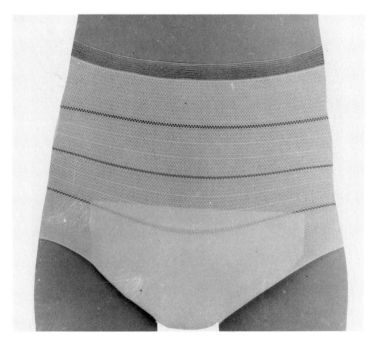

Figure 6. Tenaform Normal pants (Molnlycke).

They are all designed to have a high absorbency and to protect the rest of the bed from getting wet. The new Kylie absorbent bedsheet and the Domein 'Confidence' underpad are products worth considering.

REFERENCES

Caine M & Raz S (1973) The effect of progesterone on the adrenergic receptors of the urethra. *British Journal of Urology* **45**: 131–135.

Carlile AE, Davies I, Faragher E, Rigby A & Brocklehurst JC (1987) Aging in the human female urethra. *Neurourology and Urodynamics* **63**: 149–150.

Castleden CM, Duffin HM & Asher MJ (1981a) Clinical and urodynamic studies in 100 elderly incontinent patients. *British Medical Journal* **282**: 1103–1105.

Castleden CM, George CF, Renwick AG & Asher MJ (1981b) Imipramine—a possible alternative to current therapy for urinary incontinence in the elderly. *Journal of Urology* **125**: 318–320.

Dontas AS (1984) Urinary tract infections and their implications. In Brocklehurst JC (ed.) *Urology in the Elderly*, pp 162–192. London: Churchill Livingstone.

Fletcher TF & Bradley WE (1978) Neuroanatomy of the bladder. *Journal of Urology* **119**: 153–160.

Gosling JA, Dixon JS, Hilary OD, Critchley & Thompson SA (1981) A comparative study of the human external sphincter and periurethral levator ani muscles. *British Journal of Urology* **53**: 35–41.

Griffiths DJ (1980) *Urodynamics*. Medical Physics Handbooks. Bristol: Adam Hilger.

Hald T (1984) The mechanisms of continence. In Stanton S (ed.) *Clinical Gynecological Urology*, pp 22–27. St Louis, Toronto: C.V. Mosby.

Hilton P & Stanton SL (1981) Algorithmic method of assessing urinary incontinence in the elderly. *British Medical Journal* **282**: 940–942.

Kass EH & Brumfitt W (1978) *Infections of the urinary tract*. Chicago: University of Chicago Press.

Klarskov P, Gerstenberg TC & Hald T (1986) Bladder training and terodiline in females with idiopathic urge incontinence and stable detrusor function. *Scandinavian Journal of Urology and Nephrology* **20**: 41–46.

Lapides J (1976) Further observations on self catheterisation. *Journal of Urology* **116**: 109–171.

Malone-Lee JG (1983) The pharmacology of urinary incontinence. In Barbagallo-Sangiorgi & Exton-Smith (eds) *Ageing and Drug Therapy*, pp 419–440. New York: Plenum Press.

Moisey CU, Stephenson TP & Brendler CP (1980) The urodynamic and subjective results of treatment of detrusor instability with oxybutinin chloride. *British Journal of Urology* **52**: 472.

Phillips JI & Davies I (1980) The comparative morphology of the bladder and urethra in young and old C57BL/Icrfat mice. *Experimental Gerontology* **15**: 551–562.

Resnick NM, Yalla SV & Reilly CH (1985) Advanced urodynamic investigation of the very aged institutionalised patients: new insights. *XVth Annual Meeting of the International Continence Society Meeting, London*.

Stanton S (1984) Urethral sphincter incompetence. In Stanton S (ed.) *Clinical Gynecological Urology*, pp 169–191. St Louis, Toronto: C.V. Mosby.

Turner-Warwick R & Whiteside CG (eds) (1979) *Clinical Urodynamics, Urologic Clinics of North America*, Philadelphia: W.B. Saunders. Vol. 6, no. 1.

Wilson PO, Barker G, Brown AOG, Russel A & Siddle N (1981) Steroid hormone receptors in the female lower urinary tract. *XIth Annual Meeting of the International Continence Society*. Lund: Saogs Trelleborg.

7

Post-menopausal bleeding

HARVEY WAGMAN

Post-menopausal bleeding (PMB) is one of the most important symptoms in gynaecology, as it is frequently associated with genital tract malignancy. It is defined as vaginal bleeding following one year's amenorrhoea from the date of the last menstrual period. The age at which the menopause occurs varies widely, but the range quoted is 45–53 years. The average age used to be 47 years but is now thought to be 51 years (Tindall, 1987). Any woman who is still menstruating after 55 years should be viewed with suspicion, and post-menopausal bloodstained discharge has equal significance to that of post-menopausal bleeding. The major responsibility of the physician is to exclude the presence of malignancy in the genital tract which can occur in 5–25% of patients presenting with PMB.

PATHOPHYSIOLOGY

The post-menopausal endometrium is a thin layer of tissue in which the glands are sparse, the epithelium simple and the stroma compact. Cystic dilatation of glands lined by inactive epithelium needs to be distinguished from hyperplasia with the more complex and convoluted glands and thick cellular tissue.

Under the influence of oestrogens, the post-menopausal endometrium becomes thicker with an increase in nuclear activity, a dilatation of glands eventually amounting to endometrial hyperplasia. Progestogens are inhibitory to the proliferative effects of oestrogen and thus reduce the risk of hyperplasia. The post-menopausal woman is not devoid of oestrogen. In addition to minute amounts of oestradiol from the ovary, oestrone is produced in adipose tissue by the peripheral conversion of adrenal androgens. Thus, especially in obese women, there may be sufficient oestrogen to stimulate the endometrium.

CAUSES

A practical classification of causes is summarized in Table 1.

Table 1. Classification of causes of post-menopausal bleeding.

Genital
  Malignant
    (a) Primary tumours of the genital tract
    (b) Secondary tumours
  Non-malignant
    (a) Oestrogens
      (i) exogenous
      (ii) endogenous
    (b) Benign tumours
    (c) Infections
    (d) Injuries
Extragenital

Genital causes

Malignant

Adenocarcinoma of the uterus is the most commonly found malignancy with PMB. Some 80% of patients with carcinoma of the uterus present with PMB. The likelihood of a patient with PMB having a malignancy increases with age, approximately 15% at 50–59, increasing to 35% at 60–69 and 42% at 70–79 years (Rubin, 1987). Obesity, nulliparity, late menopause, diabetes and prior pelvic irradiation are recognized factors with an increased risk of endometrial carcinoma (Bamford and Wagman, 1972). The diagnosis can only be confirmed by histological examination of the endometrium.

Cervical carcinoma was a prominent cause of post menopausal bleeding in the past. It used to be twice as common as endometrial carcinoma, but with present cervical cytology screening and increasing use of colposcopy, the incidence is now only one fifth of the incidence of carcinoma of the body of the uterus. Any patient who has had infrequent screening is at higher risk as 90% of patients with cervical carcinoma have never had a smear. Associated factors contrast with endometrial carcinoma and include early age of first intercourse and numerous partners.

Patients with rarer gynaecological tumours may present with PMB. Carcinoma of the fallopian tube usually occurs in the 50–60 age group, and may present as a profuse watery discharge in a nullipara. Suspicions are alerted if there are no curettings at dilatation and curettage (D&C) and laparoscopy will reveal a tubal lesion.

Uterine sarcomata occur in patients aged over 60. These include low grade stromal sarcoma, mixed mullerian tumours or rhabdomyosarcomas. The uterus is symmetrically enlarged, soft and cystic. The bleeding may be profuse and at curettage a fleshy, necrotic polypoidal tumour is revealed.

Carcinoma of the vulva presents in the elderly, with a friable ulcer at the vulva. Although obvious on examination, difficulties in diagnosis may arise in obese or incapacitated patients.

Primary squamous cell carcinoma of the vagina is rare but occurs in the 60–80 year age group when an offensive discharge is associated with PMB. A friable raised ulcer is seen on speculum examination on the wall of the vagina. The vagina is also the site of secondary tumours either by direct spread from bladder or cervix, or vulva or via blood or lymphatic spread from primary tumours in the body of the uterus, kidneys or breast.

Non-malignant

Exogenous oestrogens. Exogenous oestrogens are an important and increasingly common cause of PMB. In the United Kingdom perhaps 20% of the target population are users whereas in the United States the figure may well approach 50%. Unopposed oestrogens are alleged to increase the risk of uterine cancer by a factor of 1.7–12, associated with the dose and duration of treatment (Ziel and Finkle 1976; Hammond et al, 1979; Horwitz and Feinstein, 1978). The uterine carcinoma which develops under the influence of oestrogen appears to be small, well differentiated and carries a better prognosis than carcinoma starting 'de novo'.

The beneficial and protective effect of progestogens (medroxyprogesterone acetate 10 mg daily) taken for 7–10 days in each cycle for patients on hormone replacement therapy is well established and there have been very few cases of endometrial cancer reported in these patients. Gambrell et al (1980) suggested that the incidence of endometrial carcinoma is 56 per 100 000 woman years in users of oestrogen and progestogen compared to 359 per 100 000 woman years in users of oestrogen alone. The incidence in those women not taking hormones is 248 per 100 000 woman years.

Endogenous oestrogens. Oestrogens can be detected in the post-menopausal woman. Small amounts of oestradiol are still produced by the post-menopausal ovary but the main oestrogen is oestrone, arising from the peripheral conversion in adipose tissue of androstendione from the adrenal. Endogenous oestrogen is related to body weight and the oestrogen may reach a level able to irregularly stimulate the endometrium and so produce post-menopausal bleeding.

Endogenous oestrogens can also rarely be produced by some ovarian tumours. Granulosa cell tumours and theca cell tumours are small in size and yellow in colour. Both tumours arise after the menopause and produce high levels of oestradiol with a reduction of gonadotrophins. The unopposed acyclic levels of oestrogen cause uterine bleeding, endometrial hyperplasia and even carcinoma. It is worth noting that androblastomas (Sertoli cell tumours) produce oestrogens as well as androgens and can present as a rare cause of PMB.

Benign tumours of the genital tract. This is a common yet innocuous cause of this symptom. Intrauterine polyps (adenoma), submucous fibroids, cervical polyps and vaginal polyps are common causes, and their management is easily accomplished by excision with histological confirmation.

Infections. Atrophic vaginitis (senile vaginitis) is caused by common pyogenic organisms in a vagina which is oestrogen depleted and has lost the natural defences of glycogen, Doderlein's bacillus and lactic acid. The vagina may be red and speckled or contain a purulent discharge. The condition rapidly responds to local oestrogens. Curettage is necessary as a concurrent uterine lesion may coexist.

Trichomonal vaginitis can be suspected by the characteristic odour of the frothy vaginal discharge and the demonstration of the trichomonas on a wet film. Oral metronidazole is curative. The white discharge of candida vaginitis is often associated with glycosuria. The organism can be cultured on Feinberg–Whittington media and antifungals which include clotrimazole are helpful.

Tuberculous endometritis can present as PMB—the diagnosis is made by finding the characteristic granuloma on histological assessment of the curettings.

Discharge of copious pus following D&C for PMB can occur when a pyometra is present. This is a collection of pus in the uterus which failed to drain owing to narrowing of the cervical canal for one of several reasons: carcinoma of the corpus; carcinoma of the cervix; stenosis following radium; past surgery to the cervix. Infection gains entrance to the uterus and the atrophic endometrium is converted into granulation tissue. A culture swab should be taken and the procedure abandoned once satisfactory drainage is established. Appropriate antibiotic therapy is prescribed and a repeat curettage after two weeks is necessary to exclude an underlying neoplasm.

Injuries. Lower genital tract traumata can be a source of PMB. These are often associated with prolapse, decubital ulceration in the untreated and grossly prolapsed cervix and vagina. However, when prolapse is treated by ring or shelf pessaries, these themselves can cause vaginal ulceration or bleeding. The treatment is to remove the foreign body and prescribe local oestrogens.

Extragenital causes

These must never be forgotten and the clues they may present are elicited in a careful history. In elderly and obese patients, however, it is not always possible to establish such a history.

A urethral caruncle is a red mass at the external urethral meatus: histologically it is granulation tissue, although on rare occasions it may be a true urethral polyp. These have to be distinguished from prolapse of the urethral mucosa which is oedematous, ulcerated and friable. If local oestrogens do not improve the condition, then diathermy excision is indicated. Haemorrhoids and fissure in ano may be thought to be the cause of PMB in such cases; careful examination under anaesthesia will reveal the true problem.

The serious conditions of carcinoma of bladder, bowel or rectum can present as 'vaginal bleeding' but an exact history with a careful curettage, cystoscopy and sigmoidoscopy can make the correct diagnosis. Recurrent bleeding may indicate such causes.

In a survey by Kintis and Calvert (1982) into the causes of PMB detected in 1972 at a district General Hospital in Northern England, 152 patients were submitted to curettage and the causes were subdivided into three main groups, malignant, non-malignant and idiopathic. Out of the 152 patients, 22 had malignant lesions (14.5%). These included 14 with endometrial carcinoma, seven with squamous carcinoma of the cervix and one patient with carcinoma of the ovary. 102 patients had benign lesions, mainly cervical polyps and atrophic vaginitis, and either atrophy or hyperplasia of the endometrium. In 28 patients no cause was found. Four per cent had extra-genital causes, the bleeding originating in the urinary tract. It is worth noting that at that time, approximately 5% of the population would have been using hormone replacement therapy and widespread comprehensive cytology screening for carcinoma of cervix had not been instituted.

INVESTIGATIONS

A careful history is essential regarding the length, nature and duration of the episode of bleeding. The amount and any relation to trauma as well as the persistence of the loss is of great significance. Any exposure to oestrogens, dermal patches or ointments is carefully sought and confirmation that the blood is being lost from the vagina and not from an extragenital source.

Vaginal examination is carried out in a good light when a careful inspection of the vulva, perineum, external urinary meatus, vagina and cervix is made. Both the dorsal and left lateral positions may be necessary to view the four vaginal walls. Bimanual palpation of the uterus and adnexa is performed to reveal any masses or induration of the parametrium. Cervical cytology and possibly vaginal cytology samples are taken. The vaginal sample can be used for hormonal assessment if clinically indicated, although abnormal endometrial glandular cells can be detected by this method.

In addition, specialized investigation can be considered. Serum follicle stimulating hormone (FSH) and oestradiol levels are useful in the evaluation of endometrial hyperplasia—which can occur in hyperoestrogenic hyper-plasia, in the presence of carcinoma of the body of the uterus or with an oestrogen-producing tumour. A raised oestradiol with a low FSH is found with a granulosa cell tumour but with neoplastic endometrial hyperplasia or small endometrial carcinoma, the oestradiol is low and the FSH within the post-menopausal range. In cystic endometrial hyperplasia, the oestradiol is marginally raised but the FSH is low.

The cornerstone of investigation must be, however, an examination under anaesthesia with careful dilatation and curettage. The benefit of a thorough examination with accurate inspection of the lower genital tract and external genitalia is invaluable. Any lesion within the lower genital tract can be seen, biopsied or excised. Vaginitis can be confirmed and careful sounding of the uterus is possible followed by dilatation of the cervix and fractional curet-tage. Cystocopy and sigmoidoscopy can be performed at the same time if clinically indicated by the history. The procedure is easily accomplished in many elderly patients on a day case basis under general anaesthesia, a method which is efficient, acceptable and cost-effective. In medically compromised patients, however, admission to hospital is necessary.

Although other methods of endometrial sampling on the conscious patient have been advocated, their sensitivity ranges from only 50–80% (Rubin, 1987). Whilst these methods may have a place in the screening of asymptomatic women having hormone replacement therapy, once PMB has occurred, with its high risk of malignancy, only the most comprehensive and accurate methods should be employed. It must be recognized, however, that 'office' techniques may confirm an obvious lesion and therefore save time in organizing definitive treatment.

Table 2. Office techniques for evaluation of the endometrium in women with PMB (from Rubin, 1987).

Technique	Total cases	Cancer detected	Cancers at D&C	Unsatisfactory specimens (%)	Sensitivity (%)
Saline irrigation	1251	45	64	17	70
Brush cytology	191	7	11	32	64
Vacuum aspiration	122	5	10	25	50
Jet washer	181	6	10	21	60
Isaacs cell sample	189	10	12	4	83
McMark cell sample	101	6	9	—	66
Endometrial biopsy	811	*60	62	3	96

*Four to six specimens obtained under general anaesthetic using Randall or Novak biopsies.

Even under the most favourable conditions there can be difficulties with dilatation and curettage. Problems may arise during dilatation of the stenosed or distorted cervix. Perforation is a real possibility in an atrophic or diseased uterus. The procedure should then be abandoned to avoid bowel damage or intraperitoneal haemorrhage. Immediate laparoscopy can be helpful and curettage under laparoscopic control attempted, otherwise careful consideration has to be given to an emergency hysterectomy.

Hysteroscopy allows visualization of the endometrial cavity with direct biopsy of any lesions seen. The procedure may be performed under general or local anaesthesia (paracervical block). The uterine cavity is distended with either 5% dextrose in water or 32% Dextran in dextrose. The technique is sometimes helpful but often impossible with an atrophic vagina or cervix and has therefore not achieved universal acceptance. However, Valle (1981) has reported on 134 post-menopausal patients evaluated by hysteroscopy prior to D&C. Biopsies were performed on any lesions seen and these were compared with the pathological diagnosis from later curettage. The procedure was performed under local analgesia with many patients requiring systemic analgesia. No lesions were missed at curettage when a large portion of the endometrium was involved, but in three patients with focal carcinoma diagnosed at hysteroscopy, only one was found at curettage. This technique warrants further assessment and should be considered in recurrent PMB to exclude the small focal lesion.

Ultrasound of the pelvis is steadily becoming an integral part of the gynaecological examination and may give additional information concerning unexpected pathology in the pelvis. The more sophisticated and expensive techniques of magnetic resonance imaging (MRI) and computerized tomography (CT) scans cannot be justified in the routine patient with PMB but may have a place in a difficult or unusual problem.

MANAGEMENT

Treatment is dictated by the cause. Adenocarcinoma or sarcoma of the uterus, carcinoma of the cervix, vagina and vulva are best treated by gynaecologists experienced in oncology. A mixture of radiotherapy, radical surgery and chemotherapy could well be required, depending on the stage of the lesion and the medical fitness of the patient (see Chapter 8).

Endometrial hyperplasia may be treated with progestogens (medroxy-progesterone 20 mg daily) but repeat curettage is necessary after an interval of three months. When the hyperplasia persists, particularly with the presence of atypicality, hysterectomy is indicated.

Atrophic vaginitis can be adequately managed by local oestrogens (1 gm equine oestrogen per vaginam twice weekly) or systemic HRT once the curettage has proved negative. In conditions in which oestrogen is contrain-dicated, for example carcinoma of the breast, pessaries of lactic acid NF nocte can be offered.

PMB after previous hysterectomy requires a careful examination under anaesthesia, cystoscopy and sigmoidoscopy. The most likely cause is atro-phic vaginitis but other rare causes need to be excluded. Recurrent PMB is a worrying condition for the medical attendant. It requires renewed efforts by a scrutiny of the history and a meticulous examination under anaesthesia, cystoscopy and sigmoidoscopy. Hysteroscopy, if technically possible, is useful to exclude a small focal lesion possibly missed by the curette. The procedure must be performed by an experienced gynaecologist as additional measures such as laparoscopy, or even hysterectomy, may be the only way of excluding significant pathology including the very rare tubal carcinoma.

SUMMARY

PMB is a common symptom, which is associated with approximately a 20% incidence of malignancy in the genital tract. Every effort, therefore, needs to be made to exclude adenocarcinoma of the uterus, a condition with a good prognosis if an early diagnosis is made. In most other patients the cause of PMB is minor and can readily be controlled.

REFERENCES

Bamford DS & Wagman H (1972) Radium menopause. A long term follow up. *Journal of Obstetrics and Gynaecology of the British Commonwealth* **79:** 82–84.
Gambrell RD, Massey FM, Castenda TA, Ugenes A, Rice L & Wright J (1980) Use of the progestogen challenge test to reduce the risk of endometrial cancer. *Obstetrics and Gynecology* **55:** 732–738.

Hammond CB, Jelovesek FR, Lee KL, Creasman WT & Parker RT (1979) Effects of long term oestrogen replacement and neoplasia. *American Journal of Obstetrics and Gynecology* **133:** 537–547.

Horwitz RI & Feinstein AR (1978) Alternative analytic methods for case control studies of endometrial carcinoma. *New England Journal of Medicine* **299:** 1089–1094.

Kintis GA & Calvert W (1982) Postmenopausal bleeding. One hospital—one year. *Journal of Obstetrics and Gynaecology of India* **32:** 676–683.

Rubin SC (1987) Postmenopausal bleeding: aetiology, evaluation and management. *Medical Clinics of North America* **71**(1): 59–69.

Tindall VR (1987) Clinical aspects of ovulation and menstruation. *Jeffcoate's Principles of Gynaecology*, 5th edn, pp 80–102. London: Butterworths.

Valle RF (1981) Hysteroscopic evaluation of patients with abnormal uterine bleeding. *Surgery, Gynecology and Obstetrics* **153:** 521–526.

Ziel HF & Finkle WD (1976) Increased risk of endometrial carcinoma among users of conjugated oestrogens. *New England Journal of Medicine* **293:** 1167–1170.

8

Gynaecological cancer in the elderly

CHRISTOPHER HUDSON

Nearly all the female genital cancers seen in the reproductive and early post-menopausal years are to be found in the elderly. Some tumours of germ cell origin are virtually confined to the younger age groups, including infants and adolescents. Secondary malignant transformation of a hitherto benign dermoid cyst is, however, age related, and the dysgerminoma covers the full age range. In contrast to other cancers, ovarian cancer in the elderly tends to be more anaplastic and aggressive.

TREATMENT—GENERAL CONSIDERATIONS

Surgical ablation of the upper female genital tract, including the gonads, in the elderly has few physiological sequelae. Ordinarily the post-menopausal uterus is small and atrophic and its removal is unlikely to disturb the function of the adjacent organs of bladder and bowel in the way that removal of a larger organ may do, particularly with respect to defaecation. It would, however, be chauvinistic to assume that there would be no psychological nor emotional sequelae from genital ablation in the elderly. It would, moreover, be unwise to assume that coital function has ceased in the elderly and the implications of malignant conditions which arise in or affect the vagina, either directly, or as a result of treatment, need to include this consideration.

It is clear that treatment decisions must be completely individualized and take into consideration the constitutional status of the elderly person involved. Extreme frailty may be a contraindication to vigorous therapy but the toughness of the elderly under such circumstances is often under-estimated. Of greater relevance will be the emotional status, and dementia must be a contraindication to anything other than purely palliative measures. The difficulty, of course, is that this very diagnosis in the early stages may be subjective. Obviously the views of general practitioners and other primary health care professionals will be of paramount importance in making such a decision. The views of relatives, however, need to be viewed with some caution, as they may not necessarily reflect the best interests of the elderly person concerned.

It is worth remembering that the actuarial life expectancy of a healthy octogenarian will be of at least five years and the propriety of offering therapy designed to enhance the prospect of five year survival should be seen against this backcloth. Therapeutic nihilism based on the notion that the appearance of treatable malignancy in the elderly is necessarily a terminal event cannot be justified. Each case and individual should be carefully assessed and staged, and management decided on its merits.

ANATOMICAL SITES

Female genital cancer in the elderly may be conveniently considered in four anatomical sites.

Uterine corpus

Presentation. The most obvious presentation in the elderly is post-menopausal bleeding. Except in very advanced disease, there are few other symptoms, although suburethral metastases may cause urinary problems (see below).

Investigation. A definitive diagnosis may be achieved by vaginal cytology, but a negative does not exclude the condition—the false negative rate is of the order of 50%. Histological confirmation may be achieved by aspiration curettage or full diagnostic D&C (dilatation and curettage). These procedures may be difficult in the elderly because of flexion and adduction deformities of the hips.

Pathology. Most commonly the lesion is an adenocarcinoma, usually endometrioid. The concurrence of pyometra is common in this age group and carries an enhanced risk of perforation. More rarely, sarcomatous lesions occur. Mixed mesodermal tumours with heterologous or homologous elements are particularly found in the elderly. In all these tumour types the prognosis is poor if the disease has spread beyond the uterus.

Treatment. Where feasible, abdominal total hysterectomy and bilateral salpingo-oophorectomy would be standard management. The alternative of vaginal hysterectomy (preferably with salpingo-oophorectomy) should not be over-looked as being less disturbing for an elderly person than a formal laparotomy, but requires significantly more surgical experience and expertise. Where the surgical option is to be avoided intracavitary brachy-therapy may be used, but similar problems of access have been encountered. External beam teletherapy may be desirable for more advanced disease, but the morbidity and acceptability need careful evaluation. High dose progestogen therapy is effective in arresting disease in some 25% of cases. Sensitive tumours are usually well-differentiated and unfortunately in the elderly anaplasia is the general pattern.

Cervical and vaginal

Presentation. Vaginal cancer is rare in any age group, but tends to be a lesion of the elderly. In the past there was the known association with irritant rubber pessaries, but this is less likely to be the case with modern inert plastic prostheses. Carcinoma of the cervix can present at any age. Either of these tumours may be present with post-menopausal bleeding, foul discharge and eventually fistula formation.

Pathology. In most instances, the pathology of primary tumours will be squamous cell carcinoma. Adenocarcinoma is usually of endocervical origin. When malignancy is found in the vagina and, in particular, if it is an adenocarcinoma, the possibility of it being a metastasis should be borne in mind—indeed this may be the most likely diagnosis.

Investigation. Staging is essentially clinical. Extensive imaging would tend to be academic as treatment of the local lesion is required virtually without regard to evidence of spread. Histological confirmation is essential before definitive treatment. When adenocarcinoma is found, sigmoidoscopy and barium enema are needed to exclude extension from a colonic primary.

Treatment. Morbidity is high and treatment indicated even though it may be unrewarding. Surgery has very little place except occasionally for cancer associated with a major degree of genital prolapse, for which trans-vaginal extirpation may be advocated. On the other hand replacement of the prolapse for the insertion of intracavitary sources may be followed by such local fibrosis that the prolapse does not recur. Variations on intracavitary and external beam techniques should be individualized according to the needs of the patient and the dictates of access.

The management of complications, in particular fistula formation, is extremely difficult. Abdominal diversion or disobstruction of the urinary tract is in general to be deprecated. The possibility of colpocleisis for temporary palliation should always be borne in mind as it is a relatively simple procedure to perform even though not universally successful.

Suburethral metastasis from endometrial carcinoma may respond to hormonal therapy, but is also amenable to interstitial therapy using radio-active grains or wires. If ulceration of the bladder base has occurred with fistula formation so that urinary diversion is required, radical local excision is feasible with minimal morbidity, the procedure being identified as a 'radical urethrectomy', which involves the excision of one or both inferior pubic rami in continuity with the urethra and bladder base.

Uterine adnexa

Pathology. Cancer of the ovary and fallopian tube is even less favourable in the elderly than the depressing situation found in younger age groups. With the exception of the altered distribution of tumours of germ cell origin referred to above, a full range of pathology is seen including the 'clear cell' so-called mesonephroid tumours, which are rarely seen under the age of fifty. The spectrum of malignancy covers the full range of aggression from un-differentiated anaplastic tumours to well-differentiated neoplasms of low potential malignancy. For this reason an attitude of total therapeutic nihilism to an ovarian neoplasia in the elderly is not justified and pleasant surprises do occur. Thus there would have to be very strong contraindications for an operation not to be advocated when there is a clinical diagnosis of ovarian cyst.

Presentation. The presentation of ovarian cancer in the elderly is as protean as in younger age groups. Because in this age group the disease is more often anaplastic and of advanced state, the distension due to ascites is a more prominent diagnostic feature. Ultrasound in the first instance may be sufficient to indicate bilateral adnexal disease and thus a major gynaeco-logical component.

Investigation. The definitive diagnosis is made at laparotomy. Chest X-ray and urography may be helpful. Other imaging may be desirable, however, when the possibility of metastatic disease to, rather than from, the adnexa is to be considered.

Treatment. Modern surgical management of ovarian cancer requires that a major surgical effort should be made to extirpate all abdominal disease. Occasionally this requires that an affected loop of bowel should be resected. The age of the patient alone should not be used as an excuse for avoiding such a surgical endeavour if complete extirpation could be achieved thereby. It is exceptionally rare for primary radical surgery for ovarian cancer to result in colostomy, and certainly in the elderly this should be avoided. However, straightforward resection and anastomosis of intestine is normally very well tolerated and is not a particularly hazardous or difficult procedure. In short, the criteria of operability and the propriety of radical oophorectomy are very little different in the elderly than from the younger age groups. On the other hand, over-treatment should be avoided and the need for hysterectomy needs to be determined individually in the light of local conditions. Removal of a small mobile uterus may actually simplify bilateral oophorectomy. Hyster-ectomy is certainly required if there is obvious local extension or fixity of the uterus. There is another factor, namely an association with endometrial cancer. This particularly occurs with endometrioid ovarian cancer, but also rarely happens with certain other histological types. Such a double diagnosis may be excluded by diagnostic curettage. Apart from the above consider-ations, the addition of hysterectomy to bilateral oophorectomy for ovarian neoplasia adds nothing to the operation except a measure of complexity. It is accepted that bilateral oophorectomy is the minimum surgical procedure and emphasis must be laid on the 'bilateral'. Even though the second ovary may, to the naked eye, appear totally normal, sequential involvement of a residual ovary occurs sufficiently often for this to be important.

Even if radical tumour clearance is not achievable the palliative benefits of bulk reduction by removal of the ovaries and omental 'cake' should not be overlooked. The question of adjuvant chemotherapy is more vexed. Aggressive intravenous chemotherapy is almost certainly inappropriate for the elderly and likewise abdominal radiotherapy would not normally be considered useful. However, single agent alkylating agent chemotherapy will have few side-effects and may produce a dramatic, even though short-lived, response. Chlorambucil or melphalan are ideal agents for this purpose, cyclophosphamide having the disadvantage of causing epilation, which may be particularly distressing to the elderly.

Vulval

Presentation. Cancer of the vulva is especially a malignancy of the elderly and presents one of the most difficult therapeutic problems in this age group. Disease which is advanced at presentation is common, but lethal extension and metastasis is a late phenomenon.

Although the vulva is an external site, the elderly female is commonly very sensitive concerning the pudenda and neglect of malignant lesions in the early stages is common. Pruritus is a symptom which should demand close inspection. Ulceration leading to foul discharge or bleeding is only a very late phenomenon.

Pathology. Almost all lesions will be keratinizing squamous cell carcinoma. Histological confirmation is essential as occasional non-malignant ulceration must be excluded. Rare variants of malignant pathology will not influence management.

Investigation. Other than biopsy, clinical staging is virtually all that is required. This may be difficult without anaesthesia and judgement must be used if a single procedure is contemplated.

Treatment. The natural history of the disease is singularly unpleasant. For this reason radical local therapy may be the best form of palliation. Ineffective surgery is actually worse than no surgery at all. There is no suitable chemotherapy regimen for squamous cell carcinoma in this area and external beam radiotherapy can cause quite considerable distress with a moist and sore reaction. If local excision is to be undertaken, it must be radical in the context of being wide in all dimensions. It is clearly pointless to make a wide lateral excision while skirting the proximal margins within millimetres of the tumour. Nevertheless, primary closure is obviously a great advantage and fine judgement needs to be exercised in determining the extent of an appropriate excision.

There are various options for dealing with lymph nodes, which may be adapted to the needs of the elderly. In the absence of clinically positive nodes, prophylactic radiotherapy to the groins has been used. Alternatively, a superficial lymphadenectomy may be included with a wide total vulvectomy. There is a high rate of dehiscence of groin incisions, particularly if the perforating blood vessels at the saphenous opening require ligation. The situation is aggravated by lymphorrhoea, which predisposes to infection.

In spite of the above comments an interesting development, particularly for posterior lesions which encroach upon the anal canal, is the adaptation of the combination therapeutic regimen devised for squamous carcinoma of the anal canal using both radiotherapy and simultaneous sensitizing low dose chemotherapy. The agents used for such a programme include mitomycin, fluorouracil or hydroxyurea. The unpleasant reaction to radiotherapy may be justified if thereby it is possible to preserve the integrity of the anal sphincter and subsequent continence.

In developing countries where longevity is not the rule, the surgical treatment of vulval carcinoma is one of the more rewarding areas of surgical oncology and even in the elderly appears to be extremely well tolerated. In a developed community, such surgery is sometimes perceived as over-treatment by those in attendance who may be unfamiliar with the natural history of untreated disease.

UNIDENTIFIED PELVIC MASS

The challenge of this diagnostic problem in the elderly must at all times be tempered with the best interest of the individual paramount. In practice, simple questions need to be asked:

1. Is there a benign aetiology possible for such a mass and, if so, can the diagnosis be achieved without surgery? A calcified uterine fibroid obviously has to be considered and this diagnosis may be sufficiently accurately determined by a combination of ultrasound and plain radiography.
2. Could an unidentified mass in the pelvis be due to diverticular disease? If this were the case, operation might not be indicated. As diverticular disease is common, the possibility of a double diagnosis should not be overlooked.
3. Are there any criteria suggesting inoperability, either constitutional or local? If this and the exclusion above have been eliminated, exploratory surgery should almost always be carried out. It does not matter who does the operation, provided that the surgeon can deal appropriately with genital or colonic pathology. The remarks made above concerning colostomy are particularly pertinent.

POSTOPERATIVE PAIN RELIEF AND TERMINAL CARE

Surgery in the elderly may induce confusion, compounded by the strange environment and adverse reaction to drugs. Immobility, lack of subcutaneous fat, risks of water intoxication, all make postoperative care significantly more difficult: measures such as prophylactic anti-coagulation are probably not justified as haemorrhagic complications are serious. Wound dehiscence may be a problem—mass closure with high polymer or unabsorbable suture material may be preferred to catgut.

Fears about respiratory depression or aggravating constipation may induce restriction of opiate analgesic. The cardinal principle should be that adequate pain relief should be provided even if more hazardous than in a younger patient. A sympathetic anaesthetist is a useful ally in this situation.

CONCLUSION

The need for individualization of therapy and management of gynaeco-logical cancer in the elderly is as great or greater than in younger age groups. All decisions need to be taken with total care of the patient in mind, a situation which is not always made easier by immediate relatives and well-meaning lay persons involved in the care of the elderly.

SUGGESTED READING

Weintraub NT & Freedman ML (1987) Gynecologic malignancies of the elderly. *Clinics in Geriatric Medicine* **3**: 669–694.

9

Sexuality in the elderly

JOHN KELLETT

It might reasonably be asked, what is the function of sex in the elderly? The female human loses fertility progressively from the age of thirty, if not before, and is unlikely to conceive after fifty. Therefore her youngest child is likely to be independent when she is seventy. Although the elderly continue to consume the resources of the planet without being directly 'productive', they play an important supportive function, both in the rearing of their grandchildren, and in stabilizing the society in which that child will grow.

Marital stability is still an important component of this supportive roll, and also can play a major part in the continued survival of the individuals comprising the couple. The arthritic wife may be the communicator for her deaf but agile husband, for example. The sexual drive as a means of reinforcing the pair bond is far from exhausted, but when separated from reproductive function is more susceptible to the winds of culture.

Just as food preference is induced by culture so sexual behaviour will conform to the expectations of others. Nevertheless sexual activity in old age is recognized in many primitive cultures (Winn and Newton, 1982). The mistake is to assume that what characterizes sexual behaviour in the elderly of our generation will necessarily reflect the behaviour of the elderly in the next. This is relevant in the context of cross-sectional studies which can only tell us what is happening today; they cannot predict accurately what will be happening in twenty years.

PSYCHOLOGICAL CHANGES OF AGEING

Longitudinal studies emphasize that differences between the generations are often as big as the effects of ageing; thus information from cross-sectional studies has to be treated with scepticism. Most studies are agreed, however, that ageing is associated with increasing introversion and cautiousness—highly appropriate responses of the individual to decreasing physical robustness. Social activity changes its focus from the community to the family, although total social activity tends to remain unchanged.

The making of sexual contacts is a risky business, opening the initiator to rejection and the responder to an intensity of involvement which may be too much to bear. It is often far safer to suffer in lonely isolation than to go out to meet potential partners. The strong sexual drive of youth forces the healthy adolescent into the maelstrom of dating, but the elderly depend more on their need of company to follow the same path. Whilst established patterns of behaviour and problem solving are well retained, the elderly have greater difficulties in new learning. Thirty years of life with one partner will have established modes of communication which may be inappropriate elsewhere. 'Old thing' may be a term of endearment to the long-wed wife, but not to the equally old girlfriend.

SEXUAL BEHAVIOUR AND AGEING:

By far the largest and most detailed study of human sexual behaviour was that of Kinsey et al (1948, 1954), although this too has its limitations. His size of sample in the younger age groups was sufficient to break it down into subgroups like married, unmarried, social class, etc. (2886 males and 1211 females aged 21–25), but the samples of those over the age of 60 were very small (87 white males and 39 black over the age of 60 years with only four whites over 80 years; 56 females over 60 years). One can thus only extrapolate from the effects seen in younger cohorts.

From Table 1 it will be seen that ageing is associated with a lower frequency of orgasm in males affecting all outlets except intercourse with prostitutes and other extramarital partners. The range becomes narrower. In their early twenties some couples were having intercourse 29 times a week but by the age of 60 years this fell to 3. This very wide variation may be a result of the low sample size in the elderly, however.

Table 1. Sexual activity in the male by age and marital status.

	Age	N	a		b		c		d		e		f		g		h	
			%	freq	%	freq	%	freq	%	freq	%	freq	%	freq	%	freq	%	freq
Single	21–25	1535	99	2.7	81	1.4	61	1.2			29	0.4	59	1.3	15	1.1	81	0.4
Married	21–25	751	100	3.9	48	0.5	100	3.5	100	3.2	13	0.2	24	1.3	8	0.4	59	0.2
Single	41–45	56	96	1.9	61	1.0	66	1.1			39	0.5	52	0.8	38	1.2	48	0.2
Married	41–45	272	100	2.0	33	0.3	99	1.9	99	1.6	9	0.2	24	0.5	2	0.8	54	0.2
Married	56–60	67	99	1.1	19	0.2	97	1.1	94	0.9	8	0.3	22	0.7			28	0.1

Key: N, sample size; %, reporting activity in that sector; freq, Mean number per week of those active; a, total outlets to orgasm; b, masturbation; c, total intercourse; d, marital intercourse; e, intercourse with prostitutes; f, nonmarital intercourse excluding e; g, homosexual orgasm; h, nocturnal emissions.

According to Kinsey's informants physical measures also show a decline, permanent erectile impotence affecting 0.1% of men aged 20, 6.7% aged 50, and 27% aged 70. Morning erections become less frequent, the angle of erection increases (the erect penis in the standing posture is further from the upright position), and mucous secretion is reduced.

Kinsey's data (Kinsey et al, 1953) also suggests a reduction in activity with age in the female (Table 2). With the greater likelihood of the female being left without her male partner than the reverse it is not surprising that solitary orgasms, largely by masturbation, become the more favoured means of

Table 2. Sexual activity in the female by age and marital status.

			a	a	b	b	c	c	d	d	e	e
	Age	N	%	freq	%	freq	%	freq	%	freq	%	freq
Single	21–25	2810	60	1.1			11	0.18	35	0.9	5	1.0
Married	21–25	1654	88	2.8	99	3.0	15	0.22	27	0.6	1	0.9
Ex*	21–25	238	76	2.3			21	0.32	41	1.0	6	1.1
Single	41–45	179	68	1.6			18	0.14	50	1.0	—	—
Married	41–45	497	93	2.0	94	1.8	31	0.13	36	0.6	—	—
Ex	41–45	195	84	1.8			36	0.24	58	0.7	—	—
Single	56–60	27	44	0.9			—	—	—	—	—	—
Married	56–60	49	82	0.8	80	1.3	29	0.19	35	0.2	—	—
Ex	56–60	53	55	0.6			30	0.16	42	0.4	—	—

Ex* means previously married; a, total orgasm; b, marital coitus with or without orgasm; c, dreams to orgasm; d, masturbation to orgasm; e, homosexual orgasm; %, percentage reporting activity in that sector; freq, mean number per week.

achieving orgasm with age. Between 26 and 30 years of age it is responsible for 14% of female orgasms, but at 51 to 56 it is 26%. Nevertheless, coitus remains the commonest method—78% at 26–30 and 67% at 51–55. Unlike single males and previously married females, single females were markedly less sexually active than married women.

Detailed and reliable as the Kinsey data are, they can be criticized as being cross-sectional the behaviour of 60 year olds in 1950 differing from 20 year olds not only because of ageing but because of different life experience. Pfeiffer et al (1968) in the first report on the Duke University sample of ageing volunteers, confirmed the cross-sectional findings of Kinsey but was able to show that the decline in sexual activity and interest with age was not universal. Comparing measures on the same sample of 116 subjects four years apart, 13% showed an increase in activity and 15% an increase in interest. Both partners agreed that when intercourse ceased it was the decision of the male.

More interesting is the second report from the Duke University which, unlike Pfeiffer, controlled for the effect of a live partner. George and Weiler (1981) (Table 3) studied the second longitudinal sample of elderly which (unlike the first) was not based on volunteers but on 502 subjects aged 46 to

Table 3. Levels of sexual activity (0–4 scale), 0, never; 1, <1 sexual relations per week; 2, 1–2 per week; 3, 3 per week; 4, >3 per week.

Age at start	n	Mean sexual activity (standard deviation)							
		1969		1971		1973		1975	
		Men							
46–55	63	2.03	(0.87)	1.98	(0.81)	1.95	(0.92)	1.94	(0.93)
56–65	74	1.47	(0.86)	1.53	(0.85)	1.45	(0.91)	1.32	(0.81)
66–71	33	1.13	(0.81)	1.21	(0.96)	1.19	(0.91)	1.17	(0.81)
		Women							
46–55	57	1.70	(0.92)	1.71	(0.90)	1.69	(0.88)	1.66	(0.85)
56–65	36	1.32	(0.81)	1.24	(0.89)	1.20	(1.02)	1.16	(1.04)
66–71	15	0.79	(0.83)	0.77	(0.83)	0.76	(0.91)	0.67	(1.00)

71 studied for the next six years at two-yearly intervals. 278 subjects remained married throughout, and were used for the report.

The only group to show a significant change over the six years were the males aged 56–65 (F = 4.14 $P<0.04$) though the cross-sectional data were significant throughout. Allowing for the cross-sectional data dealing with ten year rather than six year gaps there is still strong evidence that the inter generational differences far exceed the effects of ageing, in both sexes.

Kinsey et al (1953) found that sexual activity in the older female was dependent on the availability of an active partner. As women tend to choose partners older than themselves, and the proportion of males to females in older population steadily drops (Table 4) many females may give up coitus through force of circumstances. Certainly as far as married couples are concerned the cessation of coitus is usually due to the male even if this is by involuntary erectile failure (Pfeiffer et al, 1968). Continued sexual activity in the male would appear to relate to an early age of onset of sexual activity, a feeling of well being, and health, and a non-dogmatic personality (Vallery Masson et al, 1981).

Table 4. Ratio of males: females in the UK in 1985 (derived from Social Trends, 1987).

Age	Ratio
15–29	1.03
30–59	1.00
60–64	0.88
65–74	0.79
75–84	0.53
85 +	0.40

Continued sexual activity in the older female is highest in the current married, and is progressively less frequent in the divorced, widowed, and the never married (Corby and Solnick, 1980). Resumption of sexual activity in the first 14 months after widowhood is greater if the death was anticipated, if experience of extramarital coitus was present, and if the widow is younger. It is less if the previous marriage was sexually satisfying and if a strong attachment remains to the deceased (Kansky, 1986).

The most abrupt change in the female occurs at the menopause when the ovaries cease to secrete oestrogen and progesterone. However, one might expect female sexual drive to be retained if testosterone is important, as ovarian and adrenal androgen production continues unabated (see below).

PHYSICAL CHANGES

The effects of ageing and oestrogen lack are described elsewhere in this volume. In this section I will concentrate on the effects on sexual arousal, orgasm and resolution, as described by Masters and Johnson (1966). The sexual arousal phase is usually divided into the excitatory phase where the physical changes of engorgement are greatest, and the plateau phase where these changes remain roughly constant until the orgasmic phase. In the elderly, however, these two phases are much less distinct and the physical changes of arousal continue to mount until orgasm. The changes disappear more quickly after orgasm except for nipple erection.

Excitatory phase. The swelling and parting of the labia majora is rare after the age of fifty. Nevertheless some swelling of the labia minora, though less frequent and intense, may occur until the age of 60 years. Vaginal lubrication is usually delayed from the 10–30 seconds noted in younger females to 1–3 minutes and is less prolific, though particularly sexually active females may retain the response of younger women. Lengthening of the inner two-thirds of the vagina and tenting caused by elevation of the uterus are much less marked. Nipple erection is similar to that of younger females and occurs early in the excitement phase, though the later engorgement of the areolae is much less marked as is the swelling of the breasts as a whole. The response may also be asymmetrical.

Plateau phase. The skin flushing which occurs in 75% of women under 40 years during this phase is much less common. The clitoris, which does not show the swelling of the glans characteristic of the younger woman, does retract under its labial hood, and the engorgement of the anterior one third of the vagina develops as in younger women.

Orgasm. The contractions of the anterior vagina remain but whereas a young woman will experience 5–10 such contractions the older woman will have 3–5. The accompanying rectual contractions are usually absent unless the level of sexual arousal is unusually intense. Some gaping of the urethral meatus may occur but is much less frequent with age.

Resolution. This proceeds unusually rapidly in the elderly woman with the exception of the erect nipples which may remain elevated for several hours. The thinning of the vaginal lining and loss of corrugations exposes the urethra to greater risk of trauma from prolonged coitus and the elderly woman is more likely to suffer dysuria after intercourse. This and the reduction of lubrication may cause dyspareunia.

The male shows similar changes to the female. He is slower to arouse and his physiological responses are less intense. Nipple erection occurs during the excitement phase but to a lesser extent and skin flushing is usually absent. Penile erection is markedly slower in onset and often does not reach its peak until orgasm. On the other hand the ageing male can maintain his erection for longer periods without the risk of premature ejaculation. If however the older male loses his erection during the excitement phase he may be unable to regain it and goes through a refractory period similar to that of a younger man who has ejaculated.

Orgasm itself is less likely to follow arousal and is less forceful and is less clearly divided into the phases of ejaculatory inevitability and ejaculation itself. Ejaculation may occur without warning and be experienced as semen seepage rather than expulsion. Rectal contractions are absent. Testicular elevation and engorgement which are characteristic of younger males in the excitement phase is much less marked. Not surprisingly having experienced less intense physiological responses to arousal the resolution phase in the ageing male is much quicker though the refractory period will last twenty four hours or more.

DRUG EFFECTS

The needs for exercise, challenge, and sexuality are the hallmarks of the healthy individual. Ageing is associated with increasing morbidity the treatment of which, even if successful, often interferes with sexual fulfilment. Arousal in the male and probably in the female requires an intact parasympathetic nervous system and a blood supply to the penis which can increase from a resting flow of 8 ml/min to 270 ml/min. In addition, the central nervous system must be able to respond to sexual cues, and initiate a sexual encounter. It is always easier to start a treatment than to stop it and this is particularly true of drugs which are liked by the patient and remove dissatisfaction. The benzodiazepines fit this description well and are commonly prescribed. Foy et al (1986) found benzodiazepines in the urine of just over half the patients admitted to a hospital in Australia over the age of 65. Their effect on suppressing sexual desire is only now becoming recognized. The major tranquillizers are not so addictive but are equally effective in suppressing sexual drive in men.

One cannot, however, assume that a drug which reduces libido in men will do the same to women. Male sexuality is largely proceptive whilst the female is receptive. In other words the male actively seeks sexual contact and will do this without much in the way of outside stimulation. The female on the other hand will vary in her arousability to sexual overtures by the male but is much less likely to initiate them herself, especially if her potential partner is a stranger. The form of libido most associated with testosterone in both sexes would seem to be proceptive sexuality. Thus castrated males show no diminution in their erectile response to erotic films but they are much less likely to have a girlfriend (Sanders and Bancroft, 1982). Equally women with high levels of testosterone tend to show a more male pattern of sexuality. Riley et al (1987) describe high levels of prolactin as being associated more with low arousability than low interest *per se* but they confound their argument by suggesting that bromocriptine (which reduces prolactin levels) restores interest. These findings can be resolved if dopamine has a direct effect on increasing sexual interest (e.g. the increase in sexual fantasies of males treated with L-dopa) of the receptive kind, whilst testosterone increases proceptivity. This could explain why high levels of prolactin during lactation have no effect on levels of sexual activity (Alder et al, 1986; Elliott and Watson, 1985). Bromocriptine could thus increase sexual receptivity by its effect on dopamine receptors and increase proceptivity by reducing levels of prolactin.

The role of testosterone in female sexuality is in dispute (Kellett, 1984). If it is important in maintaining libido, women would have to be much more sensitive to the effects than men. However there are anecdotal but strongly held beliefs that testosterone in male replacement doses restores libido in women. Oestrogens and progestogens probably have no effect on libido but oestrogen prevents atrophy of the vaginal epithelium and thus the dyspareunia that can result from this. Hallstrom (1977), reporting on 800 women between the ages of 46 and 54, found that cessation of menstruation was associated with significant loss of sexual interest and coital frequency, although a social factor may be important as suggested by their finding that the decline was most marked in the lower social classes.

Several drugs have been implicated in causing sexual dysfunction in men including most of the drugs used to treat hypertension (Moss and Procci, 1982). However women are largely ignored in such surveys. Bauer et al (1978) studied the effects of various combinations of propranolol, methyldopa, a thiazide, and placebo in 229 women in the Australian National Blood Pressure Study and found that women were significantly more depressed and sleepy on active treatment, but they implied that there was no difference in 'sexual inclination'. Riley et al (1987) surveyed 800 patients attending the Oxford Hypertension Clinic, 22 of whom were women over the age of 60. Both treated and untreated had high levels of dysfunction only 36% reporting no difficulties with arousal and 27% were anorgasmic. Unlike men there was no difference between those on and off treatment, suggesting that drugs were not the cause of the dysfunction.

Psychotropic drugs have well-recognized effects on sexual function although these effects are better delineated in males. Benzodiazepines have been widely used as a treatment for dysfunction on the theory that most dysfunction comes from excess anxiety. It is now becoming clear that they reduce libido (Mathews et al, 1983) and the sensation of orgasm (Riley and Riley, 1986) in the female. As they are widely used as night sedatives in the elderly (Morgan et al, 1988) this side-effect needs to be fully appreciated.

The major tranquillizers like benperidol are actually promoted for their effect on reducing libido. One mechanism is by the stimulation of prolactin secretion through dopamine blockade. Dopamine itself has been found to increase sexual interest in male patients with Parkinson's disease (Bowers et al, 1971), suggesting that the blockade of dopamine may be directly responsible for the decline in libido. Major tranquillizers and antidepressants like thioridazine (Kotin et al, 1976), clomipramine (Girgis et al, 1982) and phenelzine (Barton, 1979) are used to treat patients with premature ejaculation and erectile difficulties but this is probably because they share a sympathetic alpha blocking action. Indeed they can cause anorgasmia. As loss of libido is one of the cardinal symptoms of depression, and increase of mania, antidepressant drugs are often prescribed for loss of libido. From animal work one would predict that antidepressants which potentiated 5-hydroxytryptamine would have less effect on stimulating libido than those acting on noradrenaline and dopamine. Surprisingly the only antidepressant that has been singled out as increasing libido is one of the former, viloxazine (Costanzo et al, 1982).

NON-PHARMACOPEAL AGENTS

Despite its reputation as an aphrodisiac alcohol has been shown to inhibit physiological arousal, and in the long term reduce libido. Wilson and Lawson (1976) gave women increasing doses of alcohol and measured their vaginal blood flow when watching an erotic film. They found a linear decrease in blood flow in relation to alcohol level which was evident at as low a level as 25 mg/100 ml. It also delays orgasm with self masturbation. Nevertheless its widespread use indicates its ability to increase the expectation of sexual arousal. In males it causes a reduction in levels of testosterone probably by a direct effect on the testes rather than by reduction in LH levels (Davies and D'Mello, 1985). It therefore causes a reduction in proceptivity but possibly not in receptivity, and hence its continued popularity.

Most drugs of addiction decrease libido possibly because the pleasure induced by the drug replaces the desire for sexual pleasure. Low doses may increase sexual behaviour by disinhibition whilst larger doses suppress, though opiates are more generally suppressive (Davies and D'Mello, 1985).

DISEASE

Ageing is accompanied by the changes of wear and tear and by an increased incidence of potentially lethal illness. Tuberculosis is reputed to stimulate libido (probably because the relative youth of its victims gave a spurious impression of increased sexuality) but most illnesses reduce sexual drive in balance with the capacity to satisfy that drive.

Problems arise when one partner is more sexually capable and willing than the other. Here the ladder concept of Elizabeth Stanley (1981) comes into its own. This describes how couples can satisfy each other despite being at widely different levels of arousal, through manual contact and masturbation.

Dementia is usually associated with loss of libido especially in Alzheimer's Disease. This is less true of frontal lobe dementias like Huntington's chorea, and Pick's Disease where the coarsening of personality and retention of libido can lead to disaster. In my experience retention of physical contact even without penetration is a major factor in persuading the male to continue to care for his dementing spouse (Morris et al, 1988).

Diabetes seems to spare the sexual function of the female, although Jensen (1986) found that 18% of insulin treated diabetics complained of reduced vaginal lubrication. Ellenberg (1977) studied 100 female diabetics and found, unlike the males, that neuropathy had no effect on sexual interest and orgasmic response.

Diseases affecting mobility like strokes, and arthritis may respond to simple remedies like placing a cushion under the behind of the woman, or taking analgesics an hour before making love. Here as elsewhere in old age the couple learn to alter their love-making from the frenetic athleticism of youth to gentle and prolonged caressing often without the need for penetration. Osteoarthritis of the hips may well require surgery. Where muscular weakness is the problem a water bed may help.

Abramov (1976) has recorded a high level of sexual difficulties before a myocardial infarct but even those who have continued their sexual relationship until the infarct are likely to give up, 27% stopping altogether and a further 44% decreasing activity (Papadopoulos et al, 1983), this being noted in females under 65 years. Not surprisingly the older women were more likely to stop. It has been suggested that the change is due to the fear of a further infarct and patients should be counselled to resume sexual activity when they can comfortably climb a flight of stairs. In the above study such counselling appeared to encourage continued sexual contact.

The incidence of local conditions affecting the genitalia and perineum including prolapse, and urinary infections increase with age but these are dealt with in Chapter 2 and will not be addressed here. One must emphasize however the reluctance of elderly women to complain of dyspareunia, and the doctor by failing to inquire of this symptom gives tacit support to the notion of asexual ageing. Undoubtedly some patients will respond with surprise, and very occasionally disgust, but the majority will welcome the opportunity to discuss the taboo subject.

SURGERY

The increasing skills of the anaesthetist and the surgeon have meant that age is no longer a contraindication for major surgery. As with myocardial infarction the patient may need advice about restarting sex, and appropriate analgesics after discharge from hospital. Not the least important is attention to constipation which often follows bed-rest, a change in diet, and an elderly person's embarrassment at using communal lavatories.

Mastectomy

This operation has long been recognized to produce sexual morbidity. Maguire et al (1978) found that a year after mastectomy 33% of women who were sexually active before the operation reported moderate or severe sexual problems. This was attributed to a loss of confidence in body image by the patient herself, and a negative response by her spouse. This concept has been shaken by the recent finding that the morbidity after lumpectomy is as great as after mastectomy (Fallowfield et al, 1986). Somewhat surprisingly these authors have not considered the effects of radiotherapy which was given to all the 48 subjects with mastectomy but only 34 of the 53 with lumpectomy. On the other hand the assessment was done at a mean of 16 months after surgery when the acute effects of radiotherapy would have worn off. Possibly elderly women are less vulnerable to the cosmetic effects of surgery (Jamison et al, 1978).

Ileostomy

As in so many conditions damage to the parasympathetic supply to the genitalia during removal of the rectum has obvious effects on the male in hindering erection. The effects on the female are less clear, although one would predict deficient vaginal lubrication. Burnham et al (1977) surveyed 222 women with an ileostomy, 165 having had excision of the rectum. Though a quarter of the women suffered dyspareunia before surgery and a third experienced a new discomfort after surgery, capacity for orgasm slightly increased and there was little serious morbidity. Many of the patients with Crohn's disease had experienced pain on intercourse before surgery (Brooke, 1979) and their improvement in general health may have disguised any deleterious effect on sexual function.

Spinal injuries

As in other conditions spinal lesions produce distinct syndromes in men but less clear cut ones in women. The sympathetic supply to the genitalia emerges at L1 and L2 whilst the parasympathetic emerges at S1 and S2. Since the former is largely responsible for orgasm and the latter for erection and lubrication one might expect that a lesion of the cord between these levels would block vaginal lubrication. It is certainly likely that it does block the psychogenic aspect of this response but direct tactile stimulation of the genitalia continues to induce lubrication as part of a reflex arc. Furthermore any problems concerned with the loss of this reflex can be corrected by the use of an artificial lubricant like KY jelly. Clearly lesions above the sacral outflow will abolish genital sensation and the experience of orgasm.

TREATMENT

The taking of an adequate history not only provides the information on which to base diagnosis and treatment, but legitimizes the concern of the patient and allows a private, hidden, and often guilt-ridden part of life to see the light of day. Patients may be reluctant to describe their most painful secrets on their first visit and the doctor must beware of providing reassurance on inadequate knowledge. It is essential to see the patient and her partner separately and to assure each of confidentiality if required. A male who loses interest in his wife could be having an affair, for example, neither needing nor wanting treatment, but may go through the motions to satisfy his wife.

The history should cover cultural information like the social class of the parents, their impression of their parents' marriage, and their role in the family, school and occupational record and current social circumstances, the personalities of both as seen by themselves and their partner, their previous medical and psychiatric history, and any treatment they are currently receiving; their intake of alcohol, tobacco, and other drugs; and current stresses. The sexual history should include aversive sexual experiences, ages at menarche, menopause, first date, and first intercourse and a brief account of previous partners and their courtship; life with their present partner including children, abortions and contraception; their current sexual outlets, including masturbation, fantasies and 'turn ons'. Obviously more detailed information has to be obtained about the presenting symptom including their own ideas for the cause, and attempts already made to correct it.

The examination involves assessment of their affect, intelligence, motivation, and affection for each other. If the complaint has a physical component like dyspareunia a genital examination should be performed together with a brief check on physical well-being, including pulse, blood pressure, mobility, respiratory and cardiac status, secondary sexual characteristics, blood count, electrolytes and blood sugar. Finally a note should be made of the behaviour of the couple towards each other.

Treatment is based on the notion that sexual union depends on sexual attraction followed by physiological and psychological arousal, followed by penetration and ultimately orgasm. Any attempt to cut out the arousal phase will lead to failure in the other phases. Arousal is inhibited by activation of alpha sympathetic receptors which accompanies the emotions of anxiety and anger. Often, of course, these feelings can result from sexual failures thus prolonging a dysfunction that may have been caused by something else. A way of analysing these emotional responses and to treat them is to set the couple exercises in petting limited by a ban on intercourse and in the early stages anything which can be perceived as specifically sexual stimulation. Clearly these initial limits will depend on the couple. It is helpful for the initiative in these exercises to be given to the overtly dysfunctional partner and to start by facial massage. These sessions called 'sensate focus' should last at least half an hour and occur at least three times a week (on the grounds that any lesser time will not allow time for anticipatory anxiety to dissipate.) The couple should be told to try to keep their minds solely on the sensations involved, and not to concentrate on pleasing their partner but on indulging themselves.

Couples with sexual conflicts have evolved many ways of avoiding confrontation and these mechanisms will be used to avoid the exercises. Different bedtimes and interests combine to sabotage change. The therapist may need to specify the times of the exercises in advance, emphasizing the need to do them before fatigue and drowsiness set in. Later appointments can be used to confront misperceptions, and to withdraw the restrictions. Sexual release which may be allowed at first by automasturbation in the presence of the partner can become mutual masturbation. Pain from previous sexual humiliation may lead the patient to perceive sexual advances as attempts at exploitation, rather than confirmation of her attractiveness to her partner. Resentment possibly derived from gender envy in childhood may be channelled into this one area in which some feeling can be evoked from the spouse. Such destructive perception and behaviour has to be confronted and interpreted. Each partner should be encouraged to own up to their own emotions without attributing the cause to their partner. Thus instead of saying 'You make me angry when you touch my breasts' the patient says 'I feel angry when you touch my breasts' thereby giving the partners a chance to work out why this should be.

Additional procedures include mutual examination in the clinic to remove anatomical myths, the use of vaginal trainers (phallic objects of different sizes) to enable the woman to regain confidence in her ability to accommodate a penis, a vibrator as an aid to masturbation to help her learn the type of stimulation which leads to orgasm, and the use of guided fantasy to increase the erotic perception of the partner (a woman who has received most of her sexual stimulation in the last ten years from reading romantic novels about young people may find her 60 year old spouse less appealing unless she can associate the pleasure of orgasm with his presence).

Physical remedies are more often prescribed for the male, but a vaginal lubricant or oestrogen pessaries are helpful when intercourse begins after a long gap. Testosterone injections may help a low libido but in the older woman should be accompanied by oestrogen to prevent virilization. Midodrine, an alpha stimulant may promote orgasm. Physical treatments are probably more useful when directed at physical conditions which are hindering sexual fulfilment like urinary infections, vaginitis, piles or musculo-skeletal diseases.

Over the age of eighty a significant proportion of the elderly are in institutions where they are subject to the social mores of younger staff. Double bedrooms should be available with lockable doors to ensure privacy. The dormitory may no longer be a feature of retirement homes but it is still the norm in health service accommodation, thus perpetuating the myth that only the mad and disinhibited have sex (since few normal people would make love in public.) Mixing the sexes may be the modern trend but to do this and to deny sexuality is like putting starving people in charge of a cold store, with no means of defrosting the food. Even an empty table is kinder.

CONCLUSION

The elderly woman proves to be a surprisingly flexible creature in terms of her sexuality. She can continue to enjoy orgasms long after the time that most potential partners could penetrate, but the loss of sexual activity is easily accepted. Intimate physical contact remains an important feature of bonding and the caring professions must beware of ignoring this need. This is not an area for the evangelist and a couple may need counselling as much to give up unrealistic expectations of sexuality as to continue intimate contact. Doctors are carriers of the social mores and must be careful not to transmit their own prejudices to their patients.

REFERENCES

Abramov LA (1976) Sexual life and sexual frigidity among women suffering acute myocardial infarction. *Psychosomatic Medicine* **38:** 415–426.

Alder EM, Cook A, Davidson D & West C (1986) Hormones, mood, and sexuality in lactating women. *British Journal of Psychiatry* **148:** 74–79.

Barton JL (1979) Orgasmic inhibition by phenelzine. *American Journal of Psychiatry* **136:** 1616–1617.

Bauer GE, Baker J, Hunyor SN & Marshall P (1978) Side-effects of antihypertensive treatment: a placebo controlled study. *Clinical Science and Molecular Medicine* **55:** 341–344.

Bowers M, Yan Woert M & Davis L (1971) Sexual behaviour during L-Dopa treatment for parkinsonism. *American Journal of Psychiatry* **127:** 1691–1693.

Brooke B (1979) Dyspareunia: a significant symptom in Crohn's disease. *Lancet* **i:** 1199.

Burnham WR, Lennard-Jones JE & Brooke BN (1977) Sexual problems among married ileostomists. *Gut* **18:** 673–677.

Corby N & Solnick RL (1980) Psychosocial and physiological influences on sexuality in the older adult. In Birren JE & Sloane RE *Handbook of Mental Health and Ageing.* New Jersey: Prentice-Hall.

Costanzo E, Caruso E, Germana B, Dieli G, Lamatia V & Cassarino P (1982) Variazioni della libido nei pazienti trattati con farmaci antidepressivi. *Clinica Terapeutica* **103:** 151–159.

Davies MA & D'Mello A (1985) *Drugs and Sexual Function; A Pharmacological Approach.* Harpenden: Ridge Publications.

Ellenberg M (1977) Sexual aspects of the female diabetic. *The Mount Sinai Journal of Medicine* **44:** 495–500.

Elliott SA & Watson JP (1985) Sex during pregnancy and the first postnatal year. *Journal of Psychosomatic Research* **29:** 541–548.

Fallowfield LJ, Baum M & Maguire GP (1986) Effects of breast conservation on psychological morbidity associated with diagnosis and treatment of early breast cancer. *British Medical Journal* **2:** 1331–1334.

Foy A, Drinkwater V, March S & Mearrick P (1986) Confusion after admission to hospital in elderly patients using benzodiazopines. *British Medical Journal* **293:** 1072.

George LK & Weiler SJ (1981) Sexuality in middle and late life. *Archives of General Psychiatry* **38:** 919–923.

Girgis SM, El-Haggar S & El-Hermouzy S (1982) A double blind trial of clomipramine in premature ejaculation. *Andrologia* **14:** 364–368.

Hallstrom T (1977) Sexuality in the climacteric. *Baillières Clinics in Obstetrics and Gynaecology* **4 (1):** 227–239.

Jamison K, Wellisch D & Pasnau R (1978) Psychosocial aspects of mastectomy. I: The woman's perspective. *American Journal of Psychiatry* **135:** 432–436.

Jensen S (1986) Sexual dysfunction in insulin treated diabetics: six year follow-up study of 101 patients. *Archives of Sexual Behaviour* **15:** 271–283.

Kansky J (1986) Sexuality of widows: a study of the sexual practices of widows during the first fourteen months of bereavement. *Journal of Sex and Marital Therapy* **12:** 307–321.

Kellett JM (1984) Testosterone: a treatment for low libido in women? *British Journal of Sexual Medicine* **11:** 82–84.

Kinsey AC, Pomeroy WB & Martin CE (1948) *Sexual Behaviour in the Human Male.* Philadelphia: Saunders.

Kinsey AC, Pomeroy WB, Martin CE & Gebhard PH (1953) *Sexual Behaviour in the Human Female.* Philadelphia: Saunders.

Kotin J, Wilbert DE, Verberg D & Soldinger SM (1976) Thioridazine and sexual dysfunction. *American Journal of Psychiatry* **133:** 82–85.

Maguire GP, Lee EG, Bevington DJ, Kuchemann CS, Crabtree RJ & Cornell CE (1978) Psychiatric problems in the first year after mastectomy. *British Medical Journal* **1:** 963–965.

Masters WH & Johnson VE (1966) *Human Sexual Response.* London: Churchill.

Matthews A, Whitehead A & Kellett J (1983) Psychological and hormonal factors in the treatment of female sexual dysfunction. *Psychological Medicine* **13:** 83–92.

Morgan K, Dallosso H, Ebrahim S, Arie T & Fentem P (1988) Prevalence, frequency and duration of hypnotic drug use among the elderly living at home. *British Medical Journal* **296:** 601–602.

Morris LW, Morris RG & Britton PG (1988) The relationship between marital intimacy, perceived strain and depression in spouse caregivers of dementia sufferers. *British Journal of Medical Psychology* (in press).

Moss HB & Procci WR (1982) Sexual dysfunction associated with oral antihypertensive medication. *General Hospital Psychiatry* **4:** 121–129.

Papadopoulos C, Beaumont C, Shelley SI & Larrimore P (1983) Myocardial infarction and sexual activity of the female patient. *Archives of Internal Medicine* **143,** 1528–1530.

Pfeiffer E, Verwoerdt A & Wang H (1968) Sexual behaviour in aged men and women. *Archives of General Psychiatry* **19:** 753–759.

Riley A & Riley E (1986) The effect of single dose diazepam on female sexual response induced by masturbation. *Sexual and Marital Therapy* **1:** 49–53.

Riley AJ, Steiner JA, Cooper R & McPherson CK (1987) The prevalence of sexual dysfunction in male and female hypertensive patients. *Sexual and Marital Therapy* **2**: 131–138.

Stanley E (1981) Sex problems in practice: dealing with fear of failure. *British Medical Journal* **282**: 1281–1283.

Sanders D & Bancroft J (1982) Hormones and the sexuality of women—the menstrual cycle. *Baillières Clinics in Endocrinology and Metabolism* **11**: 639–659.

Social Trends (1987) Volume 17, T. Griffin (ed). HMSO.

Wilson GT & Lawson DM (1976) Effects of alcohol on sexual arousal in women. *Journal of Abnormal Psychology* **85**: 489–497.

Winn RL & Newton N (1982) Sexuality in aging: a study of 106 cultures. *Archives of Sexual Behaviour* **11**: 283–298.

Vallery Masson J, Valleron AJ & Poitrenaud J (1981) Factors related to sexual intercourse frequency in a group of French pre-retirement managers. *Age and Ageing* **10**: 53–59.

10

Prolapse

STUART L. STANTON

Vaginal prolapse repair accounts for almost 60% of major gynaecological surgery (Lewis, 1968). With improved standards of obstetric care, smaller families and less time and physical straining in the second stage of labour it is likely that the prevalence of genital prolapse will decrease. However there may not be a fall in real numbers for some time, as the proportion of elderly rises in our population.

CLASSIFICATION

Vaginal prolapse is descent of a pelvic organ or structure into, and sometimes outside, the vagina. It is convenient to use an anatomical classification and to commence anteriorly with cystourethrocele and cystocele (which are the commonest), uterine descent, vault descent and enterocele and finally rectocele. Descent is graded clinically—slight when there is descent within the vagina on coughing, and marked when prolapse appears at or beyond the introitus. Uterine prolapse is graded to three degrees, first degree being when there is uterine descent within the vagina, second degree when there is descent to the introitus and third degree or procidentia, when the uterus is totally outside the introitus and is usually accompanied by a large cystocele.

PELVIC ANATOMY

Pelvic floor

The normal supports of the pelvic viscera are the pelvic floor muscles, pubocervical fascia and ligaments. The pelvic floor muscles are essentially the levator ani which are in two parts—the pubococcygeal and iliococcygeal muscles (Figure 1). They are covered by pelvic fascia and arise from the pelvic surfaces of the pubic bone, internal obturator fascia and the ischial spine. The pubococcygeus fans out and itself forms two parts: the anterior fibres decussate around the vagina and fasten to the perineal body and anal canal. Although anteriorly the fibres of the pubococcygeus are in close relation to the urethra, they are not structurally attached to it (Gosling,

1981). Posterior fibres join the raphe formed by the iliococcygeus muscle. The deeper muscle of each side unite behind the ano-rectal junction, to form the pubo-rectal muscle, which slings the ano-rectal junction from the pubic bone. The fibres of the iliococcygeal muscle slope downwards, medially and backwards to be inserted into the last two pieces of the coccyx and into a median fibrous raphe which extends from the tip of the coccyx to the anus. The muscle is innervated by the anterior primary rami of S_3 and S_4.

The coccygeus muscle is a flat triangular muscle arising from the ischial spine and in the same plane as the iliococcygeus muscle. It is inserted into the lateral margin of the lower two pieces of the sacrum and upper two pieces of the coccyx. It is also supplied by the anterior primary rami of S_3 and S_4. Both

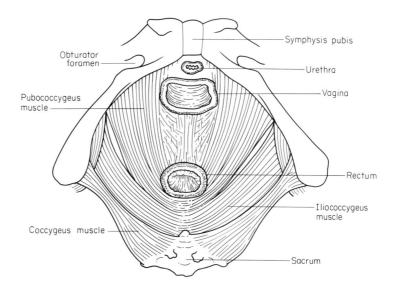

Figure 1. Pelvic floor from below—deep muscle.

these muscles act as a support for the pelvic viscera and as sphincters for the rectum and vagina. Contraction of the pubococcygeus can interrupt the urinary stream.

These muscles are aided by muscle of the urogenital diaphragm—the superficial and deep perineal muscles which originate from the ischial ramus and are inserted into the perineal body. They are supplied by the perineal branch of the pudendal nerve (S_2, S_3 and S_4) and brace the perineum against the downward pressure from the pelvic floor. The muscles are covered superficially by fascia continuous with that over the levator ani and obturator internus muscles and inferiorly by fascia called the perineal membrane.

Pelvic ligaments

These are condensations of pelvic fascia from the walls of the pelvis which support the cervix, uterus and upper part of the vagina. They include the following:

1. Pubocervical fascia, extending from the anterior aspect of the cervix to the back of the body of the pubis.
2. Lateral cervical ligaments (transverse cervical, Mackenrodt, or cardinal ligaments), extending from the lateral aspect of the cervix and upper vagina to the pelvic side walls. These form the lower part of the broad ligaments, through which nerves and vessels pass from the side walls to the uterus. The ureter passes underneath this ligament to the ureterovesical junction. The upper edge of the broad ligament contains the ovarian vessels.
3. Uterosacral ligaments, extending from the back of the uterus to the front of the sacrum. These ligaments keep the uterus anteverted.
4. Posterior pubourethral ligaments, extending from the posterior–inferior aspect of the symphysis pubis to the anterior aspect of the middle third of the urethra and on to the bladder. These maintain elevation of the bladder neck and prevent excess posterior displacement of the urethra. They may facilitate micturition and are important in maintaining continence.
5. Round ligament, which is not truly a ligament but formed of smooth muscle and passes from the labium majus through the inguinal canal to the uterine cornu. These are believed to keep the uterus anteflexed but probably play little part in supporting the uterus.

Structures involved in prolapse

A *cystocele* represents descent of the bladder through the pubocervical fascia with attenuation of the overlying vaginal skin. A large cystocele takes both ureterovesical junctions and lower ends of the ureters with it, so that these protrude outside the vagina. This can result in ureteric obstruction and ureteric damage can occur if these structures are not recognized at surgery.

A *urethrocele* is due to a lack of support of the urethra by the pubocervical fascia and posterior pubourethral ligaments; the latter are probably the most important structures supporting the urethral junction and maintaining continence.

Descent of the uterus and cervix occurs when the lateral cervical ligaments become weakened. Sometimes, particularly where prolapse is associated with nulliparity, the cervix elongates and the uterus descends without any cystocele but with an enterocele. The condensations of pelvic fascia are inadequately developed and lack their normal resilience. Prolapse of the vaginal vault follows vaginal or abdominal hysterectomy and descent occurs as a result of inadequacy of its remaining supports.

An *enterocele* usually contains small bowel or omentum and may accompany uterine descent or follow abdominal or vaginal hysterectomy or colposuspension. It used to be a common sequel to vaginal hysterectomy until its prevalence was noted and a prophylactic high fascial repair performed. Development of enterocele despite this preventive measure, may be due to the presence of deep uterovesical and uterorectal peritoneal pouches.

A *rectocele* represents weakness in the posterior vaginal wall, allowing protrusion of the rectum into the vaginal canal. The rectum descends through the rectovaginal septum and carries attenuated vaginal wall in front of it. There is separation of the posterior fibres of the pubococcygeus muscle.

AETIOLOGY

Congenital weakness of the pelvic fascia and ligaments can account for a small percentage of cases of prolapse especially where spina bifida or bladder exstrophy is present. Congenital shortness of the vagina or deep uterovesical or uterorectal pouches may also result in prolapse. However, the common causes of prolapse are childbirth and the menopause. Prolapse can occur during pregnancy. Factors said to be responsible in labour include prolonged and difficult birth, bearing down before full dilatation, multiparity, laceration of the lower genital tract in the second stage and forceful delivery of the placenta during the third stage, and inadequate repair of pelvic floor injuries. Deficiency of oestrogen at the menopause leads to loss of collagen and corresponding atrophy and weakening of ligaments (Brincat et al, 1983). This is aggravated by factors which raise the intra-abdominal pressure, namely chronic cough, constipation and heavy lifting.

PRESENTATION

Symptoms

Symptoms will depend on the type of prolapse. Discomfort is due to abnormal tension on nerves in the tissues which are being stretched and other symptoms may result from alteration of physiology of that organ secondary to prolapse. The common symptoms which are associated with most types of prolapse, are a feeling of something coming down, a lump at the vagina and low back ache which is improved on lying flat. Dyspareunia may also be present.

Cystocele and cystourethrocele. Stress incontinence may occur with just a cystocele but only if there is sufficient descent of the bladder neck. About 50% of patients with stress incontinence due to urethral sphincter incompetence have a significant cystourethrocele. A large cystocele with a normally situated bladder neck may lead to the development of a residual urine as the bladder fails to empty entirely. This is prone to infection and there may therefore be additional symptoms of frequency and dysuria.

Sometimes urgency and frequency may occur with a cystocele in the absence of a urinary tract infection. However they are not invariably due to prolapse so that when surgical correction is performed these symptoms may remain unchanged. If the patient has urinary incontinence, she may have self-induced frequency, in an effort to keep her bladder empty and so limit the severity of incontinence.

Uterine descent. This commonly causes low back ache relieved by lying flat. Third degree prolapse may cause a blood-stained sometimes permanent vaginal discharge, as the protuberant cervix is chafed during walking.

Vault prolapse and enterocele. The patient may complain of vague symptoms of prolapse. Rarely, dehiscence of a vault prolapse occurs and the patient experiences severe lower abdominal pain as small bowel is extruded through the vault. There is a danger of strangulation of bowel.

Rectocele. In addition to general symptoms of prolapse, the rectocele produces a feeling of incomplete bowel evacuation and the patient may find that digital reduction of the rectocele allows completion of bowel action.

Signs

Certain conditions predispose to prolapse, such as chronic cough and constipation. Obesity does not necessarily precipitate or aggravate prolapse (Wilkie and Stanton, 1988). To demonstrate a prolapse, the patient is examined in the left lateral position with a Sims speculum. An enterocele is distinguished from a rectocele by reducing the latter and asking the patient to cough or bear down: an enterocele may be seen or felt at the tip of the examining finger as a cough impulse. Further differentiation can be made by simultaneously examining the rectum and vagina during coughing and bearing down.

If the cervix protrudes outside the vagina, it may be ulcerated and hypertrophic with thickening of the epithelium and keratinization. Cervical cancer is not a sequel to a longstanding procidentia, but more likely to be a coincidental finding. A full pelvic examination including a rectal examination should always be performed, to exclude a pelvic mass or other condition which might cause prolapse.

Differential diagnosis

It is important to ensure that symptoms are due to prolapse and not to other pelvic or spinal conditions. A variety of conditions can mimic prolapse. A congenital anterior vaginal wall cyst (e.g. Gartner duct cyst), urethral diverticulum and a secondary from a uterine tumour (e.g. choriocarcinoma or adenocarcinoma), and a dermoid cyst can simulate an anterior vaginal wall prolapse. Procidentia may be confused with a large cervical or endometrial polyp or chronic uterine inversion.

INVESTIGATIONS

A mid-stream urine sample should be sent for culture and sensitivity. If there is a procidentia, an ultrasound scan of the kidney to exclude upper tract dilatation and a blood urea and serum creatinine are advisable. Where urinary symptoms exist, cystometry and uroflowmetry are indicated. Recent urinary symptoms and a bladder capacity of <300 ml or haematuria need cystoscopy. If frequency is dominant, a urinary diary should be completed over the course of one week.

TREATMENT

Provided there is no urinary tract obstruction or current urinary tract infection, prolapse carries no risk to life. With an older patient, medical methods are a very reasonable alternative to surgery.

Medical

A ring pessary is possibly the commonest and oldest surviving pessary in use today. Nowadays it is made of inert plastic and may be left in place for up to a year, provided that there are no adverse symptoms or signs such as bloodstained purulent vaginal discharge, which may indicate vaginal ulceration. The pessary is used to support uterine prolapse or large vault prolapse and may help a co-existent cystocele but will do little for a rectocele. It is inserted so that it rests with the posterior portion below the sacral promontory and the anterior portion placed alongside the symphysis. For extensive prolapse, the Simpson shelf pessary (Figure 2) is useful, but it is rigid and can be difficult to insert beyond a narrow introitus.

The indications for a pessary are:

1. The patient's choice.
2. When surgery is contraindicated or refused.
3. Relief of symptoms whilst waiting for surgery.
4. As a therapeutic test when there is doubt as to whether symptoms are caused by prolapse.

Contraindications are:

1. Loss or impairment of vaginal sensation.
2. Technical difficulty in inserting the pessary due to a narrowed introitus or vagina.

Physiotherapy and electrical therapy have very little role in the treatment of prolapse in the elderly.

Surgical

The surgical repair of prolapse is one of the oldest gynaecological operations

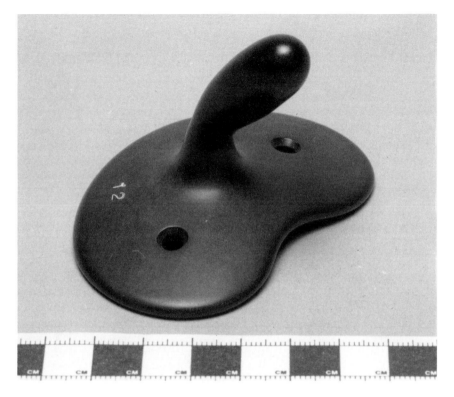

Figure 2. The Simpson shelf pessary.

having first been described by Donald in 1888 (Shaw, 1954). The majority of procedures in the elderly will be performed through the vagina. Recurrence may be corrected via the abdomen if coital function is to be preserved.

Surgery in the elderly demands careful preoperative assessment by the anaesthetist with particular attention to the cardiovascular, respiratory and nervous systems. Electrocardiogram, chest X-ray, full blood count and serum electrolytes including blood urea and serum creatinine should be standard investigations.

Procedures must be explained to the patient and relatives or carers so that all know the stages of recovery and probable time of stay in hospital. Postoperative sedation and analgesia should be light and frequent and careful assessment of day to day fluid balance is essential.

Age should not be a deciding factor in refusing surgery; rather it is a question of the patient's health and the ability of the surgeon. Surgical aims are to correct the prolapse, maintain urinary continence or correct any incontinence, and preserve coital function if that is desired. It is important to enquire tactfully about this: many older patients still continue sexual relationships and should be encouraged to do so for as long as both partners desire.

Heparinization, supportive stockings, and anti-microbial prophylaxis such as 1 mg metronidazole p.r. or 250 mg amoxycillin and 125 mg clavulanic acid (Augmentin), are used preoperatively.

Cystourethrocele

When a cystourethrocele is present without incontinence, then anterior colporrhaphy is the standard and successful procedure. If stress incontinence due to urethral sphincter incompetence is present, many of us would favour the addition of a Raz (1981) technique. Postoperative suprapubic catheter drainage is advisable.

Uterine descent

Vaginal hysterectomy rather than the Manchester operation is considered now to be the wisest approach: as well as removing the uterus which is always a potential source of post-menopausal bleeding and malignancy, the vaginal hysterectomy offers a more effective means of correcting uterine prolapse and at the same time any co-existent enterocele, which is frequently present.

Vault prolapse and enterocele

An enterocele on its own is not a common finding unless there has been a previous hysterectomy. There may be co-existent and indistinguishable vault prolapse.

If maintenance of coital function is desired, a colposacropexy (Birnbaum, 1973) is my preferred choice (Figure 3). Sacrospinous fixation (Nichols, 1982)

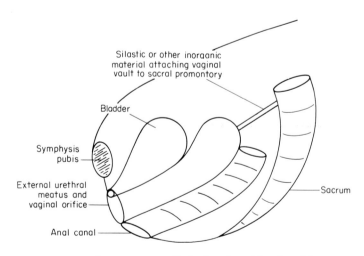

Figure 3. Colposacropexy. Sagittal section of female pelvis.

is an alternative, but I consider placing sutures around the sacrospinous ligament to be risky: it does, however, have the advantage of avoiding an abdominal incision which produces some post-operative morbidity in the elderly. If there is recurrent vault prolapse and the patient is fit and desires coital function, a Zacharin (1985) procedure may be attempted (Figure 4).

If coitus is not taking place, conventional vault prolapse and enterocele repair may be performed: the pouch of Douglas is opened, the peritoneal sac ligated and excised, and the uterosacral ligaments coapted together (usually they are very tenuous). The dissection is then widened to expose the levator ani muscles and the hernial defect is closed by a series of purse string sutures. This effectively closes the vagina.

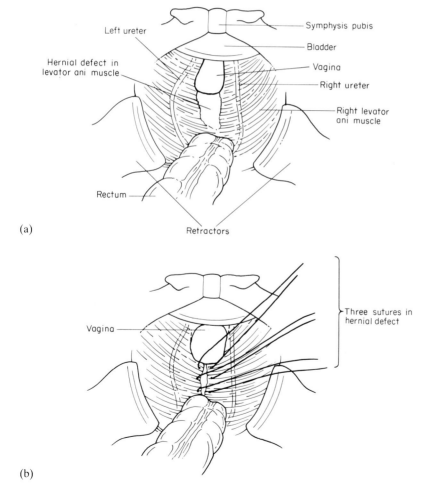

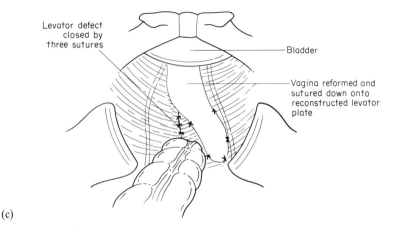

(c)

Figure 4. (a) Plan view of enterocele hernia looking into it from the abdominal cavity. (b) This illustrates the placement of three sutures in levator ani hernial defect. (c) Levator defect closed and vagina reformed and anchored onto reconstructed levator ani plate.

Rectocele

This is managed by a conventional posterior repair, but it is important again to enquire about coitus: if sexually active, adequate attention must be paid to this when performing the colporrhaphy. Postoperative suprapubic catheter drainage is wise, as micturition may be reflexly inhibited by postoperative pain.

Postoperatively it is important, particularly in the elderly, to administer carefully analgesia and intravenous fluids, and to mobilize early on to reduce the risks of chest infection and deep vein thrombosis.

CONCLUSIONS

Some cases of prolapse can be treated by conservative means. Many however will require surgery. With careful assessment and pre- and post-operative medical management many elderly patients can be treated safely by surgery. An elderly person should not be debarred from surgery for reasons of age alone. To do that is to deliberately condemn to premature infirmity an otherwise fit and independent senior citizen.

REFERENCES

Birnbaum SJ (1973) Rational therapy for the prolapsed vagina. *American Journal of Obstetrics and Gynecology* **115:** 411–419.

Brincat M, Moniz CF, Studd JWW et al (1983) Sex hormones and skin collagen content in postmenopausal women. *British Medical Journal* **287:** 1337–1338.

Gosling J (1981) Why are women continent? Proceedings of Symposium of The Royal College of Obstetricians and Gynaecologists, London, pp 1–8. *The incontinent woman.*

Lewis AC (1968) Major gynaecological surgery in the elderly. *Journal of the International Federation of Gynaecology and Obstetrics* **6:** 244–258.

Nichols D (1982) Sacrospinous fixation for massive eversion of the vagina. *American Journal of Obstetrics and Gynaecology* **142:** 901–904.

Raz S (1981) Modified bladder neck suspension for female stress incontinence. *Urology* **17:** 82–85.

Shaw WF (1954) Plastic vaginal surgery. In Munro Kerr J, Johnstone R & Phillips MH (eds) *Historical Review of British Obstetrics and Gynaecology 1800–1950*, p 372. Edinburgh: E & S Livingstone.

Wilkie DH & Stanton SL (1988) Stress incontinence and obesity: a study of the effect of obesity on urethral function. (submitted).

Zacharin RF (1985) Surgical correction of pulsion enterocele. In Zacharin RF (ed.) *Pelvic floor anatomy and the surgery of pulsion enterocele*, pp 102–133. Vienna: Springer Verlag.

Index

Note: Page numbers of article titles are in **bold** type.